DIAGNOSIS ASPARAGUS

Advocating for Assessment and Diagnosis of Autism Spectrum Conditions

CATHIE O'HALLORAN and EVA PENROSE

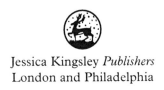

Jessica Kingsley *Publishers*
London and Philadelphia

First published in 2014
by Jessica Kingsley Publishers
73 Collier Street
London N1 9BE, UK
and
400 Market Street, Suite 400
Philadelphia, PA 19106, USA

www.jkp.com

Library of Congress Cataloging in Publication Data
A CIP catalog record for this book is available from the Library
of Congress

British Library Cataloguing in Publication Data
A CIP catalogue record for this book is available from the
British Library

ISBN 978 1 84905 535 2
eISBN 978 0 85700 957 9

Printed and bound in Great Britain

Contents

Preface

When my daughter, Eva, was diagnosed with Asperger's Syndrome (AS) in 2010 (when Asperger's Syndrome was still an official DSM diagnosis – more on that later), she and I talked about all the good things that there were about having Asperger's and about how we could explain it to people we knew. Eva has viewed the whole discussion, assessment and diagnostic process as a huge adventure and as she says 'a chance to find out more about myself.' It is important to both of us that other people have some awareness of what Asperger's Syndrome is and to view differences as just that, being *different* rather than there being a problem. One of the things we talked about soon after she was diagnosed was how we could tell others what it was like getting assessed, diagnosed and having Asperger's Syndrome. Writing it down seemed like a good way to let other people know that having Asperger's is fine, once you know what it is you are dealing with.

The purpose of this book is to share our 'journey' into discovering and living with Asperger's Syndrome with a wide audience, parents and young people. It isn't a book for professionals, and it won't tell anyone what to do or how to 'fix' Asperger's – it doesn't need fixing! Chapter 1 is about when Eva actually got her AS diagnosis and our immediate reactions. In the next few chapters we then look back at the process of assessment and diagnosis. Chapters 5 to 8 take a closer look at how the fairly abstract diagnostic criteria actually present themselves in people at the high-functioning end of the spectrum, and more specifically in Eva herself. The rest of the book looks at how Eva's diagnosis has helped us find ways to overcome the challenges AS causes, the reaction of our family and friends to her diagnosis, and looking ahead to the future.

Eva is a really positive, fun-loving person and has an incredible desire to be social and I think this is true of many youngsters that haven't got all of the 'tools' to fit in... Because of my working background as a Speech and Language Therapist, *I* am one of those tools I think, so I want to make this little book easy to read and for ordinary people, parents, carers and young people but not necessarily professionals that work with people that have Asperger's and other Autistic Spectrum Disorders (ASD). In spite of my tendency to talk incessantly (because I like to show off my vast knowledge and vocabulary!), I have tried really hard to keep the jargon and the long-winded paragraphs to a minimum. Some things are easier to abbreviate though, so we call Asperger's Syndrome 'AS' and Autistic Spectrum Disorders 'ASD'. Eva and I don't like talking about what is 'normal' either – for her, to do and think what she does is normal, so we prefer to use the term 'neurotypical' to describe behaviours, thoughts and feelings experienced by the greater majority of people who *don't* have AS or ASD.

Writing this book has been a great opportunity to get to know my daughter better and her contributions to it are the best bits, I think – Eva 'wrote' her contributions in response to me asking a very open question about each topic and then me typing (very fast!) what she said. Sometimes she would want me to read back what she had said and occasionally she would correct her grammar so all of the words that are credited to her are her own, not mine. I hope her efforts and my own can help our readers to understand AS, what a diagnosis can mean for someone who isn't neurotypical, and feel encouraged to find out more about living with and supporting people on the autism spectrum.

A Note on Terminology

Individuals are assessed and diagnosed as being on the autism spectrum by a series of observations, interviews and assessments carried out by health professionals and education specialists. The results of the assessments are measured against specific criteria for autism. The predominant set of criteria is published in the *Diagnostic and Statistical Manual of Mental Disorders* or DSM. This is the standard set by the American Psychiatric Association (APA) and is widely used throughout the world in the assessment of autism spectrum conditions. Another important set of criteria is produced by the World Health Organisation's International Classification of Diseases (ICD).

In May 2013 the DSM-5 was published, replacing the DSM-IV-R, and the diagnostic categories for autism spectrum conditions changed quite drastically. One key change is that the term 'Asperger's Syndrome' was abandoned in favour of the umbrella term 'autism' for all autism spectrum conditions. Those individuals who experience less 'severe' ASD behaviours or who are cognitively higher functioning, like Eva, when assessed against the new criteria are now likely to be told that they have 'High Functioning Autistic Spectrum Disorder' where previously they may have been told they had Asperger's Syndrome. (The ICD still includes 'Asperger Syndrome' as a diagnostic term, but a new edition, the ICD-11, is due in 2015, so who knows what will happen then.) Those diagnosed using DSM criteria *before* 2013 can make of it what they will – officially they retain their pre-2013 diagnosis, but how they choose to describe or categorise themselves is, I feel, a very personal choice. I have never been one for using a diagnostic label to describe an individual; that can only result in having preconceived ideas about what that person will be like or what they are capable of. For me, diagnostic terms are only ever helpful when they can tell me how that person is wired, what affects them (what makes them tick), and it can go some way towards telling me how they are experiencing the world. This book is a story of one family's journey through assessment and diagnosis and is intended to encourage and advocate for assessment, helping individuals to a better understanding of autism, whatever form it takes or terms used to describe it.

CHAPTER 1

Getting a Diagnosis

or 'I'm an Asparagus but I'm not green'

January 2010; memorable for everyone across the UK (but perhaps especially here in West Yorkshire) for over four weeks of deep snow, black ice, school closures and boiler breakdowns. January was more memorable still for our particular household as the month we heard the outcome of an ASD (Autistic Spectrum Disorder) assessment for our family's youngest member, Eva.

Up at 7 a.m., listening to the local radio station to the long lists of schools closed (yes, Eva's school closed *again*), roads impassable for snow, and the sensible advice to 'stay at home unless your journey is absolutely necessary'. Trouble was (and in truth, it never has been a favourite pastime of mine), I didn't *want* to be sensible; I wanted to keep my appointment at the hospital which was an 'outcomes' meeting between me and the ASD diagnostic team – a meeting I had been waiting on for some time, to hear the result of Eva's assessment. Frustrated? You bet! But determined to dig the car out if necessary, I plumped for phoning the hospital first to check that staff had made it into work.

The ASD team staff are *lovely*, including the administrative staff (who, let's face it, can be irritatingly officious at times – who hasn't, at some time in their lives, tackled an over-zealous bureaucrat on the phone, annoyingly telling us that 'the computer says "No"' or at the very least stalling and stymieing Joe Public over the phone with an over-bearing attitude?). Lucky Leeds. Lucky *me*; phoning this office always resulted in helpful, friendly, informative chats with the team admin staff and on this occasion it was no different.

I'm wondering whether or not to shovel snow, slide my way down the road and keep my 10 o'clock appointment?

Well, L has made it in, and B has phoned to say she's on her way so I'd give it a go [she says, encouragingly].

OK, tell them I'm on my way.

Less than five minutes later the phone rang:

Hi, Cathie [she has a lovely voice]. It's L, from the ASD team. I can give you the feedback over the phone if you like? It'll save you a snowy journey in?

And 11-year-old Eva is sitting at the dining-room table making 'I-know-who-that-is-on-the-phone' faces at me, and I'm scrabbling for a piece of paper and a pen so that I can make notes whilst on the phone, and my heart's sort of stopped for a few beats because I don't know how I'm going to feel, whatever they say to me. Even worse, what will Eva think and feel? I have a moment of trepidation not unlike the moment before an interview when you walk in the room with a fixed smile on your face, determinedly making a good first impression, desperately hoping that you don't trip up on your way into the room, exposing yourself to be the idiot that you feel.

So I listen, and scribble what will later be unintelligible notes on the back of an envelope, and ask a few questions. And I feel OK when she says it, put the phone down and turn to Eva and say:

She used the word 'charming' to describe you, and she says you've got Asperger's Syndrome.

Eva looks at me, grins, gives me a 'High-Five' and says:

Yey! I'm an Asparagus!

Eva (11 years)

I may be an asparagus but I'm not green. (Ha ha this is funny because 'green' has 2 meanings – the colour green and meaning someone is inexperienced and doesn't know much... I know loads of stuff!) I used the word 'asparagus' because it sounds a bit like 'Asperger's'. It's not a mistake; I am doing it on purpose to amuse myself. I like replacing the words I'm supposed to use and using words that are a bit random instead because I can picture it in my mind.

When I'd been told that I had a diagnosis I was quite excited because it was something I hadn't known about before, it told me what I was like, like horoscopes tell you what your personality is or what Chinese year you were born into...it was just another thing to describe me. I would have found out after school but because it was a 'snow day' (Hooray!) I found out earlier. Later on that day my Dad phoned to check up on what was going on because I was off school and I shouted down the phone 'I'm an Asparagus!' Mum asked me what he thought about it but I don't have a clue. I told my friends at school. They weren't really interested.

CHAPTER 2

Deciding on
Assessment

or *'they must be weird too'*

As a young girl, Eva seemed happy most of the time,
I was happy and her school was OK. To me, she
has always been my lovely daughter but plenty of
other people had commented over the years on her
'difference' to other children and I could see that some
aspects of communication and making relationships
with others could be hard for her. Aged ten, some
friendships at school started to break down and
there were instances when Eva felt bullied; a series
of events occurred that had the accumulative effect
of me wondering if she would be better off if other
people had more awareness of how she thought, how
she was wired. I never wanted Eva to have a particular
'label' to describe or explain/excuse her behaviour,

and I worried that if she did, then it would make her feel bad about herself in some way. On the other hand, she was getting called weird at school, she had difficulty being part of particular friendship groups that she wanted to be part of, and often felt excluded, and I could see that she really struggled to work out what other people might be feeling with any degree of subtlety. I think I had reached a point where I wanted Eva to understand herself and see that her 'difference' was neither good nor bad; just that – a difference. And I wanted other people to have a bit more respect for her difference, rather than seeing her as weird or quirky and consequently perceiving that as a negative. It was time to start to talk about it and find out what she really thought.

I want to comment here on what I really believe – children and young people that are not neurotypical stand out in a crowd. Childhood and education is all about fitting in, and reaching developmental norms. Individuals with AS often have their own pattern of development and do things differently from the mainstream or in their own timescale so, whether diagnosed or not, they *are* going to stand out. Having a 'label' might be useful for parents and other professionals but then we may to try to fit what we know of the child into that particular box (AS). This can be helpful or it can be limiting. What I think is useful about using the term 'Asperger's Syndrome' for Eva and other young people is that it helps them to think about them*selves*, develop an awareness of self that textbooks argue they might have difficulties with. It can give them a starting point to define themselves, rather than measuring themselves against neurotypicals, at which point they won't measure up. I think Eva sometimes feels sorry for neurotypical people because they can't see/feel/experience what she can and that's got to be good because that's the beginning of empathy (arguably absent in AS). Being aware of self is so positive – being able to say 'I'm like this' isn't about having an excuse although she did try that once, early post-diagnosis, and got verbally slapped down by her big sister very quickly:

Eva: But I need to do that because I'm autistic...

Big sister: Er, don't give me that rubbish excuse; you're just being annoying.

What I'm trying to say is that children with AS *are* different, so not telling them why, or not equipping them with a vocabulary to talk about it, makes it much harder for them to understand themselves and other people. I love it when Eva tells me 'This is what it seems like to me...' because although I have loads of expertise and knowledge of AS, I still don't know the world as experienced by her – it's all new learning for me too.

So there was Eva, at eight or nine years of age, getting called 'weird' on an almost daily basis at school and feeling confused about why she got called names. She had a long conversation with her dad one evening and between them they came up with this rationale: if someone thought she was weird, it was because she was different from them. 'Different' means two or more (people or things) that are not the same; it doesn't mean that one is 'right' and one is 'wrong'. If the other kids called her weird, it was because she was different from them – that made *them* different from her too. If 'different' could be called weird, and she, Eva, was weird, then it followed that they must be different or 'weird' too. This was really helpful to Eva; now she could articulately agree with the other kids that in fact, yes, she *was* weird and different from them, and that made them different from her too; were *they* weird as well then? So there was, in fact, no need for being called weird. Getting her head around that, I believe, is one of the main things that preserved Eva's self-esteem at that point in her life.

You might want to go back and read that paragraph again – it's really good to get your head around this explanation of how things look to Eva. Seriously, go back and read it again until you understand her reasoning; it's very logical.

Infuriatingly, it wasn't just the kids that perceived her as different. In school reports, at parents' evenings and in informal chats in the playground there were plenty of comments about Eva's 'eccentricity', 'quirkiness' or 'unusualness'. As her dad says – she 'wasn't *good* enough in school to warrant approval by the teachers and adults she came into contact with, but wasn't bad enough to get any support.' How many young people with AS are stuck out there feeling different, being called weird by the people that don't like them, and quirky by the ones that *do*, and what about the mental health and self-esteem issues that can often go hand-in-hand with AS? Especially when it's undiagnosed. So it seemed if I was going to preserve Eva's justifiably strong sense of self-worth, and raise a bit of awareness in her school population, then we needed to get an assessment and that might result in a diagnosis.

I'm going to get all preachy and soap-boxy here too – if you think your child (or an adult you know for that matter) has Asperger's or any other form of autism, and that they are reporting what Eva calls 'suffering-other-people-oppressing-me-because-I'm-different', then please, PLEASE (yes, I am shouting at this point) talk to them about autism and the process of assessment and diagnosis. It's not a bad thing. Worse, I think, to be having a hard time but unable to understand why and to end up with low self-esteem, feeling like it's all their fault but they don't have any self-awareness or understanding of how to manage their autism and so are just stuck, stuck, stuck in patterns of interaction that are dissatisfying or distressing for everyone involved.

There is a marvellous, fantastically enlightening article by one of my all-time heroes Tony Attwood about Asperger's Syndrome in girls, and how it manifests differently to AS in boys[1]... *Read* it, read it now if you have a girl with possible AS and I promise you that you will have one of those moments where a light bulb goes on in your head in the manner of a cartoon character.

Eva (14 years)

It's not that I was searching for an excuse for why I acted differently but I did need to know if there was a reason that I got left out of things and I didn't fit in. I never thought of myself as different but it just seemed that nobody was really compatible with me. I didn't question this at the time but I did feel sad about feeling left out. When my Mum talked to me about people like Luke Jackson (he wrote a book about having ASD called *Freaks, Geeks and Asperger Syndrome*[2]) and Autism and AS, I thought 'OMG (Oh-My-God) I'm like that!' There was someone I could relate to at last. Then I started thinking I AM different and then began to understand why I am who I am. For a brief time just after I was diagnosed, I had said 'This explains why I'm weird' but my Mum said 'No Eva – you're not like that because you have AS, that's just the reason you find it hard to get on with people sometimes – your personality is WHO you are and sometimes you're just plain craaaaazy.' Haha haha – she can talk!

When I got assessed and diagnosed I didn't really understand that much about AS and Autism but having a name for the reason I was different was really good. I thought it was cool but I didn't think much about what other people might feel about that and how they would react. It DID explain why I was different to other people and it made me feel special and important. So getting assessed and diagnosed is positive if you are having problems, and you feel like you don't fit in so you can get help from people. There was an interview on YouTube with someone with Asperger's so I checked it out. The presenter said – 'So-and-so suffers from Asperger's...' – which made me feel really offended. I don't think she (the presenter) had researched the subject properly because I don't think people 'suffer' from Asperger's. I definitely don't *suffer* from it now. And I definitely still have it. It's not a temporary thing.

I suppose I might have had a hard time at school when I was younger because I was isolated and an outcast in my class...my social skills weren't very good and I didn't always interact appropriately with the other kids. At the time I thought everyone else was being mean and I was an unhappy little girl. There was nothing wrong with me exactly; I just hadn't learned how to adapt who I was to suit different people. I was always the same. I was just being myself. I wasn't really doing anything totally weird or anything – I just hadn't worked out that something I said or did with one friend wasn't appropriate to say or do with the whole class. If there was a problem it was more that other kids didn't accept that everyone is different. School is a lot about fitting in with a bigger group, convincing each other that you are all the same in some way – there's lots of copying each other from what I can see; copying what they say, what they wear, what they play with. I never consciously tried to 'fit in' which I think the other kids were doing, conforming. So what I was suffering from was other people oppressing me, which may have been related to having Asperger's...but to say that someone *suffers* from Asperger's makes out that it's some kind of disease or illness, rather than there being consequences to being socially atypical.

CHAPTER 3

Getting an
Assessment

or 'gloriously gabbling on'

As a Speech and Language Therapist with a specialism in ASD, I have worked as part of a number of teams of professionals that assess children and adults for autism. Speech and Language Therapists are one of a number of 'specialist' professions that are recommended to make up an assessment team. In the UK, AS and ASD are diagnosed by a mixed group of professionals, called a multidisciplinary team. This team usually consists of (amongst others) a Paediatrician, a Speech and Language Therapist and a Clinical and/or Educational Psychologist that all see the child for assessment. Not everyone that is assessed gets a diagnosis because autism is a complex disorder and can be present in people with severe learning disabilities. However, often individuals that have severe learning disabilities are at very early levels of communication and social development. That can *look* a bit like autism to the untrained eye. In the UK, the process of assessment, what professions contribute to the team and what diagnostic tests they use varies around the country. Go further afield (as I have) and you will find that in the USA and Australia, paediatricians sometimes make unilateral diagnoses and this is hugely influenced by the financial Government support that is attached to diagnosis. Take, for example, my recent job in Melbourne, Australia, in a School for children with learning disabilities: there are large numbers of children there that are 'autistic' (a paediatrician says so) as the families of autistic children benefit from financial support from the Government and can potentially receive up to 6,000 Australian dollars a year. Many of these 'autistic' children are *not* in fact autistic but might have had limited interests and displayed repetitive behaviours as part of their learning disability. To be diagnosed with autism, children need to have difficulties with communication and interaction that are *not* at a level with their overall cognitive ability. And the DSM–IV for AS is more specific too: children need to fulfil a specific criteria that includes 'no evidence of language delay'. Let me tell you, Eva certainly didn't have any delay in language development. I'm a Speech Therapist, for goodness sake; I would have noticed.

I have home videos of Eva's second birthday, unwrapping presents and singing happy birthday to everyone – like any other toddler, she hadn't quite worked out that we were supposed to sing it to her. She was clearly commenting on her presents and asking questions, taking conversational 'turns' and responding and behaving just like any other two year old. Except perhaps she *was* a little more articulate, the vocabulary a teensy weensy bit 'precocious'. At two years of age AS is hard to identify because children are learning at a 'normal' rate; developing language skills. Higher level communication skills are learnt later in childhood, including learning non-literal language and how to make inferences from language, developing social imagination, and reciprocal communication. Lots of young children do an awful lot of 'butting in' and missing the point so, often, children with AS don't appear that 'different' until they are at a level where language and social function suddenly becomes more complicated – that's when they get 'left behind'.

To go through an assessment I needed to find out who and where the multidisciplinary team was in my local health authority and ask my GP (general practitioner) to make a referral to this team. In Leeds, the CAMHS team is the team that assess for autism. CAMHS stands for Children and Adolescent Mental Health Services and is usually an NHS service. My GP asked some questions but I pretty much rang him up, said I thought my daughter might have AS and gave some examples of why I thought that. I'm fairly confident that me saying things like 'I'm a Speech and Language Therapist with a specialism in autism and she fulfils the DSM criteria for AS' had something to do with it being so straightforward. I'm not so naive to think other parents had similarly easy routes; in fact, I *know* as many have told me (in my role as Speech and Language Therapist) that they have had to 'fight' for their child to get the assessment and acceptance of a diagnosis. Unhappily, that's what they become stuck in; a pattern of fighting for their child when they no longer have to, which alienates other professionals who find them demanding or aggressive. I'm all for fighting though...I do love a good crusade.

In spite of the ease of referrals, one paediatrician's examination, one screening questionnaire by a member of the CAMHS team and then two assessments and interviews later, plus a school screen, it took over a year from the point I picked up the phone to my GP to the snowy day in January to when Eva became officially 'an asparagus'. We were relatively lucky. I have been part of teams where referral to diagnosis took on average two-and-a-half years...

Most UK assessments include an interview with a parent. This bit is great...you get to talk about your child to people that really want to know what s/he's like. Isn't it great to be able to brag about your kids? Isn't it really sickening when you hear other people do it about their perfect offspring but we, as parents, really want to do it about our own? In an interview with a professional, you can describe all the things you love most about her, all the things that worry you, and all the time, you are being prompted and encouraged by highly skilled adults to tell them as much as possible. I came out of that bit of the assessment feeling like my kid was the greatest, most marvellous kid on the planet. (Duh! Which she obviously *is*, of course...)

Depending on the age or other characteristics of your child, they will be asked to undergo a 'play'-based assessment. Children are presented with a variety of toys and play activities and their responses are noted down; for example, to assess a young child's ability to understand that pointing indicates a direction in which to look, one member of the assessment team points to an exciting toy in the corner of the room. Children that understand this non-verbal bit of communication will turn and look in the right direction. Many children with AS do not understand such gestures and may look at the outstretched hand, or carry on looking at whatever they were looking at before. With older children or young adults the assessment may take the form of an interview with them. Eva's assessment was conducted by a Speech and Language Therapist and a Clinical Psychologist. I wasn't in the room at the time (I was gloriously gabbling on about how amazing she is in another room being interviewed by another member of the team). Eva remembers being offered some play items but preferred talking and I think she really enjoyed being asked questions, being given scenarios and talking uninterruptedly for over an hour. Of course, while the questions and conversations seemed to flow to her, she will have been carefully scrutinised by one of the assessors for behaviours related or not related to ASD, such as use of gesture, understanding gestures, using facial expression, understanding eye pointing, understanding non-literal language, and observations about what she likes and what she likes to talk about. With older children and teens they are often asked a series of questions about their relationships with other people, and what they aspire to. The assessors also look for a young person's ability to show interest in other people, for example by introducing a topic about themselves. Individuals with AS, although able to talk brilliantly about themselves and their own interests, may not pick up on clues to switch the topic of conversation if it goes on too long, or ask the assessor about *their* interests.

Schools are usually involved in assessment processes, either formally or informally questioned (there are a number of useful assessment question-naires for schools), or visits by team members to observe the child in a school setting. For teeny tiny children, they may be visited at home to observe behaviours. It all depends on where you live and how autism assessments are set up in your local authority. I have to say I feel vindicated by the assessment results (and I know this is mean spirited of me) but one of

Eva's teachers swore she 'didn't have ASD' – she had 'worked with children for years and Eva definitely wasn't autistic, just annoying.' This teacher was probably also blaming me and Eva's dad for being genetically or parentally deficient in some way. Yeah, trust me, depressing as it is, the parents often get the blame for any perceived deficiency in their child.

Often there are long waiting lists for assessments but that's not a reason to not go for it. It's also important that you consider what it will feel like to be told your child is *not* autistic or doesn't have AS. I considered this for a very long time and I think ultimately that I thought an assessment could at least give us really detailed information about Eva's skills and abilities, strengths and weaknesses. It did that very well and it is useful (and reassuring) as a parent to be told that your child has skills in one area and difficulties in another – even if, in your heart of hearts, you already know it. It's useful because you can start to talk to your child about things that are hard for them – for Eva, the thing that was hardest for her was not knowing why other people said she was weird. Once we started talking about that, it allowed me to really listen to her, really pay attention to what she was thinking and to give her some information and sometimes suggestions for alternative ways of doing things. I guess if she hadn't been diagnosed, we would still have had some really good information and would have been able to talk about 'neurotypical' behaviour in the same way, with an understanding that, whatever she was, she was not neurotypical! This has become part of our everyday vocabulary and I think it's a really useful term – it describes the 'expected' behaviours of someone and is, in fact, a stereotype and there are millions of kids out there that don't have AS or ASD but who aren't neurotypical. Hmmm, I think I shall make it a short-term mission to get this word into the everyday vocabulary of the population. It's so much nicer than being called 'weird.'

Eva (13 years)

My assessment was something I enjoyed; I felt really comfortable with my assessors. They were really nice to me. From what I can remember, I didn't play with any toys but they did ask me what I would do with certain things… I can't remember much else except having loads of fun…they asked me what games I liked to play and when I was thinking about my answer they asked me about charades and I got really excited at the thought of playing charades.

Looking back on the assessment, I think they were just trying to see how my mind worked…how neurotypical I was…for example, could I stretch my imagination? I had some ideas at the time that they were trying to find out if I had AS or not but I didn't think about the reasons they introduced certain topics or that they were 'watching' me for anything in particular.

The really good thing about the assessment, the exciting thing was that it made me feel important that I might have something that nobody else I knew had. The thought of having AS made me feel relieved...that I wasn't a freak like a lot of people made out I was, it gave me an excuse for the way I acted. Without knowing the reason why I was the way I was, I wouldn't have been able to deal with it, I would have been an outcast all over again.

It's really important for people with AS to know they have it, because otherwise they will be really confused about why things go wrong for them and then they can learn how to deal with it, how to learn to be more socially aware.

CHAPTER 4

Some Details about Diagnostic Criteria

or 'why Harry Potter would tie a pair of knickers to Hedwig's leg'

In 1988, Dustin Hoffman and Tom Cruise starred in Barry Levinson's film *Rain Man* about an autistic man and his relationship with his smooth-talking brother (Tom Cruise). The film was loosely based on a real-life autistic man called Kim Peek and won four Oscars as well as bringing autism to the notice of a world-wide audience. Asperger's Syndrome is a form of autism: the National Autistic Society (NAS) say that it is 'a lifelong disability that affects how a person makes sense of the world, processes information and relates to other people'.[3] Films like *Rain Man* or the Discovery Channel's 'My Shocking Story', where Dustin Hoffman or some genius two-and-a-half year old computes extremely large numbers in his head like a computer but can't tie his shoe laces, have raised public awareness of autism but there is still so much to learn as autistic ability is very individual. What I know about autism and Asperger's Syndrome is based on the work that I do as a Speech and Language Therapist: I have worked with children with autism for nearly 20 years and most of the young people that I work with are better-looking than Dustin Hoffman (although some of them *do* like to talk all of the time with an American accent, even in West Yorkshire – not a particular fan myself of a Yorkshire accent, so perhaps it's just a matter of enjoying how it *feels* to say words in different ways). The young people I work with always appear to me just to be 'wired' differently and don't usually have computer-brains or special talents, apart from the all-important one of simply being able to be themselves. What *I* notice about the children I work with is that they often have interests and things they like to do that are 'different' in some way. But dig a little deeper to find out *why* they do them and they generally make sense.

When Eva was diagnosed, professionals assessing children for AS or ASD using DSM criteria carried out observations and assessments that looked at three areas or domains:

1. Difficulties with social interaction

Difficulties in a number of non verbal behaviours (eye contact, using gestures, facial expression, body language) *or*

Difficulty developing peer relationships

or

Not seeking to share enjoyment or interests with others

or

A lack of social reciprocity. This means appropriate responses to others' behaviour, for example responding to friendly overtures from another person by being friendly back, or 'reading' clues from other people and behaving in accordance. A good example of this is not knowing that if someone is hurt or upset, then comforting them is a way of showing a reciprocal emotion.

2. Difficulties with social communication

A delay in spoken language developing

or

An inability to keep conversations going

or

Repetitive language

or

A lack of imaginative or social play.

3. Restricted repetitive behaviours

'Obsessive' interests

or

Inflexibly sticking to routines or rituals

or

'Stereotyped' or repetitive motor mannerisms (flicking fingers, twiddling fingers, rocking backwards and forwards)

or

A preoccupation with parts of objects.[4]

Before 2013, children needed to score at least six items from this list including at least two items of difficulty in section A, social interaction, and at least one each in section B and C with difficulties with communication and repetitive behaviours.

In 2013, with the publication of the DSM-5, the areas of difficulty were reduced from three to two (1. social communication and interaction, 2. restricted, repetitive patterns of behaviour, interests or activities), but the two new domains generally include the same features as the three old ones.

I guess I've never seen Eva as a child with a 'lifelong disability' or, for that matter, in spite of being a fairly academically bright kid, as a child with a particular talent but can see that she thinks and notices and reacts in an individual and unique way a lot of the time. Words, for example: she's always paid huge attention to words and tries really hard to work out meanings. As she's got older, she has begun to understand the ambiguity of words and language and this is both a source of annoyance for her, and amusement at times. She seems to particularly like the sounds of some words and notices similarities between them. Calling Asperger's Syndrome 'Asparagus syndrome' (or Asparagus for short) is typical; both words have the same consonant sounds and variants of vowels and syllables and, to Eva, it is just simply amusing to replace one word with a similar-sounding one. She understands the meanings are different and this is where the humour lies. It's a subtle and intentional misuse of words, not a mistake in choosing the wrong words, which is called a malapropism. I see this interest in vocabulary and language manifest itself in many ways with other young people I know with Asperger's or autism. Part of the diagnostic criteria for Asperger's has included having: 'formal, pedantic (concerned with formal rules and details) language' and 'impairment of comprehension including misinterpretations of literal/implied meanings'.

For neurotypical people the meanings of spoken (and written) language can be worked out from context, by making inferences and looking for clues in the *whole* phrase. For example, take Lewis Carroll's nonsense rhyme 'Jabberwocky' with the lines – 'Twas brillig and the slithy toves did gyre and gimble in the wabe...' This can be deciphered or decoded to some degree by our knowledge of how English language is structured. Take 'slithy toves', for example: using 's' at the end of words signals plurality in English so we can infer that 'toves' are nouns – items or objects of some sort. To describe an object, we use adjectives before the noun and thus 'slithy' is probably a descriptive term. 'Gyre and gimble' is preceded by 'did' so our knowledge of English language rules tells us that these words indicate an action of some sort. Lewis Carroll's book is full of fanciful creatures so from this context we can, in our mind's eye, put our English grammar knowledge together with the context of the whole book to work out that the Jabberwocky is talking about some other imaginary creatures moving in a lively way. Individuals with autism and Eva, on the other hand, will consider words separately and not necessarily use the context of them within the whole phrase to work out what they mean. Eva has, over the years, amused and intrigued me by her questions and comments about words. Take for example, the following:

Age 4 – *I've got a really good vocabulary because I know the word 'vocabulary.'*

Age 8 – *Does 'hypothetical' mean you're hyperactive and pathetic at the same time?*

Age 12 (whilst reading Harry Potter) – *Does 'thong' mean anything other than 'knickers'? [Big*

sister answers.] Oh good, 'cause I wondered why Harry
(Potter) was tying a pair of pants to Hedwig's leg.

So for Eva, her interest in words, their similarities or
peculiarities is her trying to make sense of what she
hears and reads, just like any other child, including
neurotypical ones! Eva is bright enough to know
(and I've been telling her for years) that people
don't mean what they say, that messages have to be
decoded by using the clues in the way they are saying
it, by the situation in which it is being said and so on.
Think of 'hitting the roof' or 'pulling your socks up'
or even 'letting the cat out of the bag'. A neurotypical
person can generally use the situation to work out the
meaning but individuals with AS may find this type
of language very confusing or even alarming. Eva's
interest in and the humour she finds in words lies
in the *individual details* of language, rather than in
decoding the message in the context of the situation.

As the end of the chapter is looming, I would like
you to think and consider one young man with AS
that I knew; please, think about what he was *hearing*,
and what he understood to have been said, not what
you know was meant by the following comment.
He looked absolutely horrified when an adult said
to him (remarking on how tall he had grown): 'Oh
M, you've grown another foot since I saw you last.'
This young man looked quickly at the bottom of his
trousers to see what had apparently miraculously
appeared there. Imagine his confusion between what
he could see and what he heard.

Eva: (15 years)

AS and ASD has got to be something different in your head...people with AS must see and experience things differently to other people but I guess if I was talking to someone with AS the first thing that I would probably notice is that their language is different, the style of talking; I'm not sure if it's an accent or intonation – we always use correct grammar and enunciate words perfectly. There are certain trends in slang and language people my age use, often textese where there's loads of abbreviations and me, personally I start out using these to mock them (like LOL or Yolo (Laugh Out Loud / You Only Live Once). I originally use these as a sort of private joke but then get addicted to using them over and over. There's something really funny about using 'street' language formally, in a posh accent – it's ironic really. Off subject slightly, thinking about the board game 'Monopoly' which has got to be the most controversial title in the history of titles – as 'mono' means 'one' and 'poly' means multiple so I find *that* really funny too.

In Year 7 and 8, people used to say I sounded posh because I didn't have a Yorkshire accent, although I grew up here and my family do – maybe this is because I'm conscious of how words are spelt and how they would sound in a dictionary definition, so that's how I say them...and I think I can sound very formal sometimes. I pay attention to grammar and enunciating words correctly – it's just something I do. I can't explain it! When I was younger I used to really like learning new words and made an effort to use complicated words when I was talking, and I've always had a good memory for vocabulary.

People with AS seem to have a mechanical way of thinking, it's always logical and it doesn't seem easy for them to 'read' other people. I think people with AS can come across as very opinionated and that can make other people react with hostility. When I was younger I felt much more that I *had* to have things the way I wanted them and would be very inflexible but I'm not like that anymore. I *did* used to be very bossy with other people and I used to be really aggressive with other kids if they didn't act the way I thought they ought to.

There was some point in time when I started to become more aware of myself, perhaps in Year 6 and 7 in school, when I started to find out more about AS and I started to question myself a bit because I knew I had AS…I was trying to fit in socially.

I'm not organised enough to have set routines that I have to stick to so I don't really relate to that stereotype of someone with AS and I don't go around saying inappropriate things any more. I think I figured out how to see things from other people's point of view, particularly trying to be sensitive and not hurt their feelings. I feel like I'm being a better person by looking at things from other points of view. It's got easier with practice but I think I work harder than most people at social situations because I consciously want to succeed at them.

I often drift off from situations and think about other subjects or put my attention on things that are unconnected and then try to make connections between things. Often my connections between things aren't obvious (to other people) and make me come across to other people as distracted, not paying attention or as my music teacher recently said look like I... 'grew up with the fairies.' Maybe these are the things that make me someone with AS.

CHAPTER 5

Social Communication

or 'So how was your day?'

Individuals with an AS or ASD diagnosis often find social communication difficult. At nine years old Eva famously learnt that a good way of starting a conversation was to say 'How was your day?' to my partner Jimmy. He would come in from work and she would bounce up and down, dying for some attention from him. Eva used to flap her arms when she was excited and pull a goofy face. This was a repetitive, stereotypical behaviour that she engaged in for a lot of years and one of the things that some children found amusing and entertaining about her. It was also something that less charitable people found 'weird'. We used to call it 'Goofing and Flapping' and I could see that it was an excited-to-see-you-but-don't-know-how-to-start-the-conversation-off behaviour. I suggested to Eva that she might want to think of something to say instead of goofing and flapping and we came up with a few possible conversation starters between us. It was great when she started saying, 'So Jimmy, how was your day?' The trouble was he'd answer her and she wouldn't know how to carry on the conversation so that after a minute of uncomfortable silence, she'd say again 'So then, how was your day Jimmy?' This could go on for three or four times before someone would crack and scream 'Aaaagh! Say something ELSE!'

Social communication difficulties mean that many children with AS don't know how to start or end a conversation and can go on…and on…and on….and on…completely failing to pick up on non-verbal signs and body language (including bored yawns) that the other person is trying to change the subject, end the conversation or just escape. Literal interpretation is also a feature: everyday language is peppered with ambiguities and this can be difficult for a person with AS to always understand. Eva and I bumped into an old friend at the exit barrier of the railway station a few years ago.

Oh L, how lovely to see you! What have you been up to?

I've just had a baby [says L, glowingly].

What? On the train? [gasps Eva in disbelief].

And of course we adults laughed, thinking she'd made a very quick and witty joke. Her interpretation of 'just' was the same as you'd find in a dictionary: 'immediately', 'now', 'in a minute'. She couldn't adapt her knowledge of the word to having a baby whereby 'just-had-a-baby' could mean in the last week, month or more.

Social communication difficulties mean that individuals find it hard to express themselves emotionally and socially. Look at this list of possible difficulties that people with AS may have with 'reading' other people too. For example, they may:

- have difficulty understanding gestures, facial expressions or tone of voice

- have difficulty knowing when to start or end a conversation and choosing topics to talk about

- use complex words and phrases but may not fully understand what they mean

- be very literal in what they say and can have difficulty understanding jokes, metaphor and sarcasm – for example, a person with Asperger's Syndrome may be confused by the phrase 'That's cool' when people use it to say something is good

- struggle to make and maintain friendships

- not understand the unwritten 'social rules' that most of us pick up without thinking – for example, they may stand too close to another person, or start an inappropriate topic of conversation

- find other people unpredictable and confusing

- become withdrawn and seem uninterested in other people, appearing almost aloof

- behave in what may seem an inappropriate manner.

And Eva did have difficulty with social interaction, in spite of *wanting* to be incredibly sociable and enjoying the company of other young people. So although she has friendships, and is chatty and communicative, she does occasionally (but, when younger, *much* more frequently):

- start conversations off by saying something completely random to another person, some of which can be deemed 'inappropriate'

- find others confusing and is unable to work out how to behave in some circumstances

- seem aloof and disinterested in some group situations.

And this makes it hard to maintain relationships.

I would like to report, though, on successes: at 14 Eva has such a huge repertoire of conversation starters, she looks like she has better social skills than many of her neurotypical peers – she will greet, hug, join in, smile, and ask questions to show her interest in others whereas some of her school mates are crippled by teenage angst and shyness or just that gauche awkwardness of being 14.

Eva (14 years)

Starting conversations off the right way has always been hard for me even though I have been getting better and really trying to practise. It depends who I am with, but with someone I've never met before or been introduced to and it might be useful to get to know them, I would feel really awkward and have no idea how to start the conversation but I suppose after minutes of awkward silence I might start off a topic about feeling awkward and not knowing what to say. I think usually when I am trying to start a conversation with someone I know well, if I can't think of something to say I would ask them how their day is going or what they are going to do at the weekend. I know that asking people questions about themselves is a really good conversation starter. Ending a conversation is difficult unless you're walking out the door shouting 'Bye!' at someone. Sometimes I know that I am going on and on a bit but feel like I have to say it all or my head will explode or something...if I see a film or read or good story I can never just summarise it for someone but have to tell the whole thing in detail

– I've got really good at noticing people's eyes glazing over!

My Mum just read me what she had written about me Goofing & Flapping and I can't remember why I found it so fun – it just seems so stupid now and the goofy face with my teeth sticking out of my mouth that I pulled was the reason I had chapped lips all the time. It's kinda making me cringe just thinking about it.

I don't think I've ever had difficulty understanding facial expressions or tone of voice except when somebody says something in a very dry humour way – but I think other people find that hard too…and I have a very dry sense of humour at times so people might find me hard to 'get' at times as well. And just for the record, I was joking about the baby on the train although Mum and I never agree on that one.

CHAPTER 6

Social Interaction and Social Imagination

or 'a perfectly good squirrel'

I have always to some extent known that Eva has AS and a part of that is that she had 'limited' or different social interactions. By this, I mean she sometimes failed to work out what other people may have been thinking or doing. A few years ago, Eva loved to play on an interactive internet website called 'Club Penguin' and often arranged to 'meet' school mates on it at a given time. If they couldn't or didn't keep to the pre-arranged time, Eva would get mad at them in their absence and needed to be given a set of explanations for why they had not kept to the agreed time. I became adept and creative in my 'excuses' for her friends:

- She's probably having her tea.

- I bet she's doing her homework.

- Her mum's made her clean the guinea-pig out.

- The computer's not working, etc.

It was hard for Eva to guess these things for herself. It just seemed to her that if S had *said* she'd be on Club Penguin at 4.30, and she was *not there*, then she was being *mean*. That was the only, single reason she could work out. This is the reality of having difficulties with social imagination. It often means that children with AS can't put themselves in other people's shoes and possibly can only work out one plausible reason for someone else's actions. It doesn't mean that Eva (or other young people with AS) is not 'imaginative' in a general way; in fact, she is actually brilliant at creating fantasy worlds, fabulously complicated artistic sculptures and games of make-believe.

To further explain what is meant by having difficulties with social imagination, people working with individuals with AS or autism use the term 'Theory of Mind'. This is an important part of a diagnostic assessment. Theory of Mind explains how for many people with autism, it can be extraordinarily difficult to put oneself in another person's shoes in order to imagine what that other person might be thinking or feeling. Simon Baron-Cohen, the Director of Cambridge University's Autism Research Centre, describes Theory of Mind as 'being able to infer the full range of mental states (beliefs, desires, intentions, imagination, emotions, etc.) that cause action. In brief, having a theory of mind is to be able to reflect on the contents of one's own and others' minds'.[5] Baron-Cohen used a term for lack of Theory of Mind that he called 'mind blindness'. People working with individuals with AS or ASD believe that mind blindness is present in all people on the autism spectrum to some degree. For those individuals on the autism spectrum with high intellectual abilities, it is possible to build some 'mind-reading' abilities through social skills training.

A simple assessment of Theory of Mind generally involves two adults being present, showing a child where something (a doll or toy) is hidden, for example, in a box. One adult goes out of the room and the remaining adult removes the toy from its hiding place and shows the child a different place where the doll is then concealed. Careful questioning of the child follows to find out where the child thinks the person that has gone out of the room will look. A neurotypical child over the age of five years will generally have 'Theory of Mind' and will know that the other person *doesn't know* what s/he knows, and will therefore look for the doll in its first hiding place. Individuals that have difficulty with social imagination, and lack Theory of Mind, will say that the person will look for the doll where it is hidden now, because that child is unable to 'imagine' himself in that person's position.

In my experience, it is possible to 'teach' these skills to young people with Asperger's very successfully although they may only be able to use these skills in some situations. Eva, for example, has got really good at thinking about what other people are thinking, feeling or doing but still continues, like many teenagers, not to be able to apply these skills to looking for 'lost' items. Sounds familiar? For example, when looking for her glasses, she can only look in the place that she knows she last put them (the kitchen unit). She would find it hard to 'imagine' that her big sister, mum or a friend would have come into the kitchen to prepare food, and cleared the unit (including the missing glasses) and have 'tidied' them away into another room. Eva will return again and again to the spot that she put them in!

My favourite 'story' about a young person lacking social imagination was told to me by a psychologist colleague of mine; whilst walking across a green and leafy playground with a young man with AS, admiring the trees and the sunshine, they saw a number of squirrels running about on the grass. One had been particularly resourceful and scampered into the bin, presumably in search of discarded apple cores or other delectable detritus, at which the young man remarked: 'Look at that! Someone has thrown away a perfectly good squirrel.' Why else would it have been in the bin?

Eva (14 years)

If you have telepathy it's really easy to work out what other people are thinking, but I don't have telepathy so I have to work these things out for myself. I used to think the only reason for people to not do what they said they were going to do, was that they had forgotten to do it. That is quite hurtful. Once I had a huge hissy fit because one of my friends just disappeared off 'Club Penguin' with no explanation. When she told me the next day that her Mum had called her for her tea then I thought that was OK but I can't remember if I could have worked that out for myself.

Now I still get annoyed if people are unreliable, for example not replying to my texts and it takes them a day to respond – *but*…I imagine that the battery has gone, or that they are out with someone or busy in some way and haven't got time to respond. I can also imagine that they have just forgotten to reply to a text because I do that, get distracted by something but I no longer just think they are ignoring me. I know that I can never really know what their situation is. I think it's taken me quite a long time to learn that. I think maybe kids that don't have AS work all that stuff out when they're little, say five or something. It's taken me a lot longer.

CHAPTER 7

Sensory Preferences and Other Stuff

or 'brace yourself for the bullet points'

Since 2013, the way people are assessed for ASD includes more emphasis on sensory behaviour. This is fantastic news because actually for children with AS, their sensory experiences are a major source of distress to their parents! I speak from experience and with great feeling on this subject. So I'm going to do the boring stuff now of explaining what 'sensory preferences' means.

Receptors all over our bodies pick up sensory information. This is called 'stimuli'. Hands and feet contain the most receptors. This information is transmitted to the brain that helps us understand and react to the sensory information. For example, if our hand touches something hot, the receptors in our hand send a message to our brain that says something like 'bloody-hell-that-hurts-quickly-move-your-hand-away.' Most of the time, we process sensory information without actively thinking about it. The sensory information we receive is through seven senses, which are sight, sound, touch, taste, smell, balance ('vestibular') and body awareness ('proprioception').

People with AS and ASD process sensory information differently to neurotypical people. This might be the greatest understatement of the 21st century (or at least in this book) and if you know someone with ASD things will start to click into place for you if you didn't know this stuff before. The problems that are caused by experiencing sensory information differently to neurotypical people are called 'sensory integration difficulties'. I am going to present you with a big, long list and numerous bullet points (I do so love a good bullet point) before I tell you a little bit of stuff about Eva's sensory integration difficulties. Forgive me the indulgence of the bullet points please, and if you really can't bear it, just skip to the next chapter.

If someone is extremely sensitive to a particular sense, this is called hypersensitivity. If they are under-sensitive, it's referred to as hyposensitive. (Check the spelling; it's a subtle spelling difference but a very conspicuous difference in experiences.) So hypo- or hypersensitivity applies to the following (brace yourself for the bullet point list):

- Hyposensitive sight

  ○ Objects can appear dark or indistinct.

  ○ Central vision is blurred but peripheral vision is quite sharp.

  ○ Poor depth perception, which can cause things like problems with throwing and catching.

- Hypersensitive sight

  ○ Objects and bright lights can appear to move around.

  ○ Images may be seen in fragments, rather than a whole.

  ○ Details are easier to focus on, rather than the whole object.

- Hyposensitive sound

  ○ May not notice or react to particular sounds.

  ○ Might enjoy particular loud sounds, noisy places or the sound of banging doors and objects.

- Hypersensitive sound

  ○ Noises can be magnified and sounds become distorted and muddled.

- Particularly sensitive to sound and can, for example, hear conversations in the distance.

- Inability to cut out sounds – notably background noise, which often leads to difficulties concentrating.

- Hyposensitive touch

  - Likes being squeezed and holds others tightly – needs to feel this tight squeeze before there is a sensation.

  - Has a high pain threshold which may result in self-harming, like biting your own hand.

  - Enjoys heavy objects (e.g. weighted blankets) on top of them.

- Hypersensitive touch

  - Being touched by others, even lightly, can be painful and uncomfortable.

  - Dislikes having anything on hands or feet.

  - Resists brushing and washing hair because head is sensitive.

  - Only likes certain types of clothing or textures.

- Hyposensitive taste

  - Likes very spicy foods.

- ○ Eats everything – grass, paper, soil. This behaviour is called *pica*.

- Hypersensitive taste

  - ○ Some flavours and foods taste too strong and overpowering. This will restrict diet.

  - ○ Some food textures cause discomfort; some children will only eat smooth foods like mashed potatoes or ice-cream. This will restrict diet too!

- Hyposensitive smell

  - ○ Some people have no sense of smell and fail to notice really bad stinks (including the smell of their own body)!

  - ○ Some people may lick things to get a better sense of what they are, because they are not getting enough information from smell alone.

- Hypersensitive smell

  - ○ Smells are experienced as intense and overpowering. This can make using the toilet difficult!

  - ○ Dislikes people with distinctive perfumes, shampoos, etc.

- ○ Can recognise people and places by their smell.

- Hyposensitive to balance (vestibular system)

  - ○ Needs to rock back and forth, swing or spin to get some sensory input.

- Hypersensitive to balance (vestibular system)

  - ○ Difficulties with activities like sport, dance, skipping, cycling, etc., where we need to control our movements.

  - ○ Difficulties stopping quickly during an activity.

  - ○ Experiencing car sickness.

  - ○ Difficulties with activities where the head is not upright or feet are off the ground.

- Hyposensitive body awareness (proprioception)

  - ○ Stands too close to others, because it's hard to measure the proximity to other people and judge personal space.

  - ○ Hard to move around rooms and avoid obstructions.

  - ○ Might appear 'clumsy' and bump into people.

- Hypersensitive body awareness (proprioception)

○ Difficulties with fine motor skills: using fingers to manage small objects like shoe laces.

○ Moves whole body to look at something.

Congratulations if you made it to the end of my list without nodding off, by the way, but all children (and adults) have *some* sensory preferences. The difference between having sensory preferences and having difficulty *integrating* sensory information is what makes neurotypical people different from those with ASD. I am fairly confident that you know a child, or you yourself, who likes the feel of a particular blankie or soft toy, and isn't it relatively 'normal' to have one as a 'comforter' at around the age 12 months to four years? It is perfectly acceptable in our society for children to use some kind of sensory preference as a comfort at that age, but we do seek to wean them off it as they get older. I suppose that is because when the child is out in public and insists on hauling the thing round with them everywhere until it is tatty, smelly and really rather grubby, Mum becomes slightly ashamed that you still love the hideous and frankly unhygienic object that was once blankie/ snuffle/woofly-bear. Sensory preferences like these do not really cause long-term problems, but when an individual has difficulty with, say, hypersensitive touch then the feel of fabric next to your skin is uncomfortable or unbearable. This is why some kids can become a bit obsessive about a particular pair of underpants and continue to want to wear them even though they are tight and a bit threadbare. Or the feel of clothes is just too much and it feels better to be naked. Many children with AS and ASD have difficulty with integrating sensory information about their body temperature so will wear big woolly jumpers in the middle of summer, or T-shirts in the snow.

Suffice to say, Eva has some sensory integration difficulties of all kinds but they are mostly private and I don't want to tell the whole world about them. I'm only mentioning it here so you get the idea. The one I *will* share with you was the day she found a hat in the school playground, picked it up because it looked a bit like one her dad had been wearing, sniffed it and then confidently put it in her pocket because it smelled right, and 'just like Dad'.

The most reported-upon sensory difficulties can be to do with food. In fact, there are a whole load of issues around food that are all sensory before you even get to taste it. Think about the smell, the texture, the temperature, the look/colour. It can all be 'wrong' before it's got anywhere near being eaten! I am sounding like Master Chef I know, but it is true that children with AS often get labelled as 'picky' or 'fussy' eaters.

Being sensitive to particular sensory sensations can impact on other things too, like attention span that can be distracted by something sensory. Visually stimulating, especially shiny things like

CDs, semi-precious stones, and glass prisms can all be sensory distractions for children with AS. I know one child who will walk back and forth in front of the window at school because he notices (and likes) the reflection of light on the glass window pane. With hypersensitive sight, the sensory information this boy is getting from the glass has become so distracting that it gets in the way of interacting with and enjoying other people.

I'm not in denial. I really like a lot of the children and young people that I work with and, although it is not politically correct to say so, I am often vastly amused by their perception of the world and their insights and observations that are so completely different from mine. Several years ago, I worked in an ASD unit in a mainstream school and discovered an eight-year-old boy that had the unnerving habit of lying on the floor by people's feet, whenever anyone new came into the room. I asked him why he liked being on the floor and he said with such feeling: 'Mmm 'cause feet smell lovely, like custard.'

I don't think that this is a particularly challenging behaviour for an eight-year-old to do that – it may be something he wants to modify as he grows up, but let's face it, there are plenty of *forty-eight*-year-olds out there with foot fetishes (and worse). He was obviously getting a lot of enjoyment from his actions but couldn't understand why anyone else would see it as strange. I could (and do) listen to Eva for hours without ever thinking she is strange in any way and sometimes wonder at a society that makes it hard for some of these amazing young people to be part of it.

Before I finally take a break and hand over to the person that really knows this stuff, think about what being hypersensitive to touch means if you are having your hair cut, brushed or washed...and what shiny lycra sportswear might be like...what about having your toenails trimmed? Parents of children with AS often report that hair washing and trips to the hairdresser are a nightmare. All of these everyday occurrences can be tortuous hell for someone with a sensory integration problem. I'll shut up now.

Eva (14 years)

When it comes to smells I always notice them more than other people, maybe because I'm more observant of the environments I'm in, and there's some smells that I find really comforting, especially if I'm really tired. A lot of people think that some smells are totally disgusting but I don't think there are smells that I find particularly horrible, just ones that I'm more tolerant of than other people – like dog poo for example – it just annoys me rather than disgusts me 'cause it's a smell that shouldn't be there. To be honest, I think the sense that influences me most is vision...if I was eating something and smelt something gross whilst I was eating I would notice it's gross but it wouldn't bother me or make me stop eating like it would some people but when

SENSORY PREFERENCES AND OTHER STUFF

I visualise what someone is saying, now *that* really grosses me out; the other day at lunch, these girls were talking about needing to go to the toilet and this really affected me and made me want to stop eating – I had a vision of what they were talking about in my mind!

I hate filing my nails because it just feels so weird that I can't do it, and so I end up biting the edges of my nails. I don't like washing my hands in school because there is nothing to moisturise my hands with and I hate the feeling of dried out skin. I can't touch things when my hands are dry – they feel disgusting.

I have some sensory traits now that I kinda feel uncomfortable talking about because I don't want them to be seen as issues; they don't stop me doing anything that I want to do or affect my family and friends in any way. I want to call them 'sensory traits' rather than 'issues' or 'difficulties' because that's a more positive way to talk about them.

CHAPTER 8

Repetitive Behaviours

or 'repetitive behaviours...repetitive behaviours...repetitive behaviours'

I think this is a really interesting element of AS and autism to write about. Repetitive behaviours mean any regularly and repeated behaviour that doesn't serve an obvious function. These behaviours vary wildly from self-harming behaviours such as banging one's head, to twiddling or flicking objects, to playing 'obsessively' on a computer game. Of course these behaviours are present in people who *aren't* autistic too – remember that to fulfil the criteria for AS and autism that there need to be other factors present, not simply repetitive behaviours.

Repetitive behaviour doesn't only mean physical activities like rocking or hand-flapping but can also mean that children and individuals have a very restricted range of interests; the stereotypes are boys that 'obsess' over Thomas the Tank Engine or dinosaurs or Doctor Who but I think these are just as motivating and likely to cause high levels of interests in neurotypical children. I think the difference between being very interested in a topic or activity and having a 'restricted interest' is that it can cause distress to the individual if someone or something interrupts their ability to talk or do whatever it is they are 'fixed' on.

Let's face it; we all have things that are of particular interest to us and that we can become 'obsessed' with. Personally, *I* indulge in many repetitive behaviours: eating chocolate, biting my nails, fiddling with my hair. These things don't serve a particular purpose except perhaps as a sort of stress relief, an unconscious attempt to 'soothe' myself. This, I think, is the most important issue that we need to consider about repetitive behaviours in people with autism; they *do*, in fact, serve a purpose: they soothe and comfort and reduce stress and anxiety and are of course, incredibly necessary if, as an autistic person, you find the world a confusing and unpredictable place. For people with AS and autism, the world is full of sensory information, conversation and situations that include people and places changing rapidly that can result in feelings of anxiety. Therefore, indulging in a repetitive behaviour makes the world a much more predictable place to be. If the behaviour involves flicking or twiddling with an object, and you have done it a squillion times before, then you *know* exactly what is going to happen to that object and you can focus your attention on it. In this way, repetitive behaviours serve an incredibly useful function; they may soothe someone who is stressed and anxious. I am a great believer in letting that person do whatever it is they need to do in order to feel less anxious.

Over the years, Eva has 'obsessed' (her words, not mine) over many different topics. She was fascinated by stars, galaxies and the universe when she was much younger and could name obscure cosmic features, she has spent hours (no – weeks) researching paganism as she grew a little older and she does tend to have a particular interest that she totally immerses herself in for weeks on end, ignoring all the other things available to her, but I do believe that these 'restricted' interests serve a purpose and are, indeed, an autistic 'strength'. I know many young children with AS who are self-taught on their topic of interest and their knowledge of their favourite subject far outstrips the knowledge of the adults around them, let alone their class mates.

Eva likes to talk about some of her repetitive behaviours as 'OCD' (Obsessive-Compulsive Disorder) tendencies to describe what she needs to do to feel less anxious. I'm not sure that I think using this terminology is OK, and I suppose that I do worry that using this term serves to trivialise the extreme anxiety and distress of people that suffer OCD. I know that Eva uses it as she sees that there is a general understanding of OCD that is reasonably positive. For example, it can refer to having a compulsion to clean or tidy and these habits are generally seen in a positive light. Talking about 'autistic repetitive behaviours' or having 'restricted interests', on the other hand, is harder to understand and explain, and I suppose Eva and I could add it to our list of things we want the world to know! For more information and a proper understanding of OCD see the MIND website.[6]

Eva (15 years)

On a larger scale I don't feel the need to constantly keep everything in order. For example, my bedroom is borderline chaos! On the other hand, I do have a compulsion to put some things in order, especially things like packs of pencil crayons that I like to put in colour sequence. Doing things like that feels a real treat and I feel really satisfied when I do it. The things that I feel like 'fixing' or ordering tend to be small scale things like stacking bowls in the kitchen cupboard or shoes that I line up. I get a bit bothered if I'm not able to do it, say it might be someone else's stuff for example. But when I get the chance to, it's so visually satisfying. Perhaps lots of people do these things but the order that I like to put things in is specific to me, like putting my clothes in the order of the thickness of the fabric...

I think when it comes to topics that really interest me, I do loads of research so I'm really well-informed and know what I'm talking about. I can spend weeks or even months researching what I'm interested in...I love 'Google'! Over the last couple of years I've been obsessed with anime (a particular genre of Japanese movie and television animation); I've watched a lot of anime, drawn lots and read loads of 'manga' (Japanese comic books). As a result of this I know a little bit of Japanese and researched Japanese terminology so I understand what I'm reading better.

Using the term 'OCD' is really highly accepted among my friends and it gets used on YouTube all the time. People use it to explain their behaviours, and use it really casually but I don't know enough about OCD to know if we are wrongly stereotyping but telling someone that I need to be autistic would be seen much more negatively.

CHAPTER 9

AS in the Family

or 'being Pollyanna'

OK – this is my chance to have a bit of a whinge… If you've read this far I am sure that at times you've been vastly irritated by my glib optimism and 'Pollyannaish' approach to living with a young person with AS. Do you remember Pollyanna? She was first written about in 1913 by Eleanor H. Porter and the story was later made into a Disney film starring an Oscar-winning Hayley Mills in the 1960s. Pollyanna was a fictional American child experiencing catastrophic life events, not least of all being lumbered with the truly awful dual name of Pollyanna, and whose story culminates in a near fatal road accident that left her crippled but who none the less found something to be 'glad' about in every dire situation. Her unrelenting optimism rubs off on the miserable and dissatisfied cast of characters transforming them from grumpy old codgers into a happily fulfilled and cheery community. Ah, dear little ginger-haired, pig-tailed and snub-nosed Pollyanna – definitely a founder member of the Church-of-Unreasonable-Cheerfulness that I have, on many occasions, been accused of devotion to.

So in spite of my tendency towards endless optimism, the reality of being a parent to *any* child is that we can suffer oppression at the hands of other parents. We are judged – for being too liberal, too strict, too lax, of 'spoiling' our children – and having a child with AS makes us particularly subjected to oppression. Eva appeared to have an overwhelming confidence at an early age, which left her able to walk into new situations including a first day at school aged four-and-a-half without so much as a backward glance whilst other children were being prised off their parents' legs and howling for the duration of their first morning in the Reception class. Other parents explained *their* child's behaviour to me in a way that appeared to me to be justifying it in some way, such as how 'close' their child was to them, implying that Eva and I lacked some miraculous and magical parent–daughter bond. This couldn't be further from the truth. I *love* Eva, and Eva *loves* me – we do indeed have a magical mother–daughter bond – no lie.

Returning to the topic of that first day at school, the simple reality was that I had told her she was going to go to school for the day so that is exactly what she did; she did not 'imagine' what that day would be like without me, or feel awkward in the company of new people. She just got on with the situation. In fact she has a fantastic ability to live 'in the moment' and especially when she was much younger could just talk to anyone or go anywhere without any inhibitions. This included talking to the parents of her class mates who quickly noticed that she was 'outspoken' and this was often judged to be inappropriate; I would watch as their faces showed confusion and sometimes disbelief when my four year old was telling them 'I like your shoes' or most memorably, when picking her up from a friend's house after school, when Eva had told the child's mother 'I'm getting a bit fed up with you telling me to sit down all the time.' She is nothing but unrelentingly honest at all times but I do have to add that she was never invited back to that particular child's house again.

So parents judge other parents. That's the reality of life and having a child that is not neurotypical makes other parents even more judgemental in my experience...and I want to whine about it a bit. (Feel pre-warned – you can skip this chapter if you really can't bear a bit of self-indulgent grumbling.) I have often felt excluded and so has Eva because she did not 'fit in' with other parents' ideas of what my child should be but it really didn't help her or me to be oppressed in this way, and in the long term, is it good for other kids too, to only be faced with people that all act the same? Where do they learn tolerance and patience or how to be positive role models for others if they are not trying to include other people in their experiences?

Of course there are practical things that make living with AS in the family hard work, not least of all Eva's hypersensitivity to food textures: instead of sitting down to relaxed family meals I find myself slumping over the dining table exhausted from cooking two meals – one for the family and one for Eva who really used to struggle to try new foods or textures. And then there is the constant checking and checking again that she has understood what I am talking about. It's hard work making things explicit! In terms of her understanding of the world and social situations when Eva was younger, I really had to make sure that I was being precise and accurate about planned events – 'just a minute' never worked. Even as she got older, I feel that I was helping her over and above the usual amount as a parent to organise herself and this included me working very hard at supporting friendships as she *always* needed help with thinking of things to do with her friends rather than leave them to simply 'play' together.

I'm lucky that my knowledge and experience as a Speech and Language Therapist helped me with working out which bits of AS were unproductive (like 'Goofing and Flapping') and providing her with alternative behaviours. It's helped me to understand something about her sensory traits rather than just feeling frustrated at some behaviours. I guess the bottom line is that being a parent is hard, but being a parent of a child with AS is a different challenge that perhaps there is less understanding and support for. It probably isn't easy for the child either, or their other family members – I have persuaded Rosy, my older and very neurotypical daughter, to contribute here, as I think her feelings and experiences of living with someone with AS could be very different from mine as a parent.

Rosy (26 years)

Having a sister with AS is normal, 'cause I don't know what having a sister without AS is like...I don't see her as somebody with a great big label on her head, she's just my sister and she's great. I love her to pieces and there are loads of great things about her. She's really, really funny; quick and witty and has a sense of humour like nobody else I know – she can be quite obscure at times and that's hilarious...with some people that are witty I often think 'I wish I'd thought of saying that', but with Eva I know I would NEVER have thought of saying what she says because she's so original. I think there is a stereotype of someone with AS – male, geeky, obsessed with Star Wars and able to play the piano really well but Eva isn't any of those things – she's a clever girl and knows lots about The Simpsons and Dr. Who, she's gorgeous looking, amusing and very loveable… It's made me realise that you can't have a stereotype and that all people are different whether they have AS, ASD or not. I'm definitely more tolerant of people that are 'different' in some way since I learnt about Eva's AS – it's made me more accepting of other people and I get annoyed by other people's intolerances. I wish our society was more focused on an awareness of autism in the same way that our society supports us to and demands that we be more tolerant of religious, cultural, political differences; I think there are a lot of people out there being treated badly because of autistic differences… I've met adults with AS and my awareness of AS has helped me understand how they are operating, why they are acting the way they are and not taking their attitude or apparent lack of interest in me personally. I think I've learnt to interpret behaviour more widely; rather than just seeing someone as 'rude' I may see that they don't have the communication or interaction style to conform to what is my idea of 'polite' behaviour.

Eva (14 years)

Mum just asked me to write about what it's like living with neurotypical people but I must say that I don't think that I live with neurotypical people – for a start there's a higher ratio of pets than people in this house – guinea pig, piggy-shaped cat, goldfish and the dog…but I think I'm living with a Mum that's completely nuts, and so is my sister. That isn't to say that they share any features of AS as far as I know.

The reason I was so weird when I was little, wasn't necessarily because of my AS but because my family are totally (to quote my mother) 'banonkers' – a cross between 'bananas' and 'bonkers.' Well, actually I know that I *did* have some weird things that I did, like 'goofing and flapping' and banging my wrists together when I was little but that was how I expressed myself and hadn't worked out that it didn't conform to what other people did when they were excited. I was never bothered by people's reactions really – but I didn't like being called names at school.

I vaguely remember being frustrated by my Mum who used to seem patronising but I know that she was trying to help me live more easily with people who didn't 'get' me…I still get frustrated with her when she points out traits I used to have but don't have now and when she tells me what I did – also, she doesn't like me to have my own angle on things and we don't always agree….and she often doesn't get my sense of humour.

I loved having Rosy around as a big sister and there were always a big group of her female friends around the house that I used to call 'The Sisters' (it's a joke). I think her friends are fantastic and I seem to get on with them really well…I always feel like when I've spent time with Rosy and her friends that they're great role models but I used to act around my friends the way she did with hers, and that wasn't always appropriate because I'm 11 years younger than she is. It's definitely easier now we are both older... for a 4 year old to act like a fifteen year old is totally inappropriate I think, but the gap between what we are interested in and what we do isn't as wide now.

CHAPTER 10

Sharing the News

or 'being an ally for Asperger's'

Once Eva had a diagnosis, I thought carefully about who we would tell and what we would say. Obviously, I had discussed it with (some) family members and friends and told them the outcome of the assessment as soon as I had it. I had also told Eva's (new) high school that she was undergoing assessment and asked for the assessment report to be copied to school. Doing that was about getting support for myself as well as Eva; it allowed me to talk about Eva with school as she had an identifiable 'problem' that they wanted to know about so they could work out how to support her best. If I'm brutally honest, having the AS 'label' was a bit like saying 'told-ya-so' to some people who had found it hard to interact and get close to Eva when she was younger. I let Eva decide if she wanted to tell her friends, and mine as well as family members. My brother, Kevin, and Eva have always got on well – she's always been close to him and he has shown unswerving bias in her favour since she was tiny. I think that's been because she never had some of the inhibitions that children can have around adults, but has always chatted to him endlessly (to his amusement) and his ability to listen attentively to her has made it a mutually satisfying relationship! I think it probably also had a lot to do with 'bonding' over 'Doctor Who' Christmas specials and both of them having ridiculous senses of humour. I asked Eva did she want to tell her uncles, aunts and grandparents and she said she didn't mind if I told Kevin – his reaction was fantastic! He said: 'So what? She's just brilliant' and that was the end of *that*.

We may have talked about it in the ensuing years but it has never been an issue for anyone in our family; my extended family and friends are as interested in Eva as they have ever been, and don't treat her any differently and haven't changed in their approaches to her as far as I can see. Without harassing my relatives and friends and conducting an interview on 'Attitudes to Eva – before and after' I guess I just have to trust my own judgement and say that it is of interest to them to find out a bit about AS but that none of them feel any different about Eva because of a diagnosis.

I have to start a special, shiny-new paragraph to sing the praises of Eva's high school. She started high school without a diagnosis and her teachers there have, from the very start, generally been positive and supportive of her, actively encouraging her in many ways and concerned that she is happy in school. I do believe, though, that actively having a diagnosis of AS has helped the school staff to understand her, and perhaps lessened some of the frustration they may have experienced over her. Look at it from a teacher's point of view – you see a pupil that is capable of average or above-average academic achievement in most subjects, but who often appears not to have listened, or not to have understood, or not to have been organised enough to complete work, ask questions, ask for help and generally appears ditsy and on another planet...*that's* got to be frustrating and I know of at least one teacher this year that voiced his frustration about Eva not asking for help when she needs it, and being disorganised with school equipment. I think that irritation is a result of not clearly understanding how the communication process breaks down for Eva sometimes; understanding AS and some of the communication difficulties associated with it, such as finding it hard to make inferences, is really important in school life and teachers benefit from understanding this.

Recently, Eva was told to go to a particular room for an exam at a particular time. When she got there, the door that she routinely went through was locked so she hung about in the corridor wondering what to do, and thinking she had made a mistake about the time. Eventually she wandered back into the main school building only to be accosted by a teacher frantically searching for her. 'Where have you been?' was the frustrated demand to which Eva replied that she had gone to the room and the door was locked. 'But you were supposed to go in through the *back* door' the exasperated teacher cried. How was Eva to have worked that out? It was outside of her previous experience and although she did know that there was another entrance to the room, she hadn't used it herself before in spite of the teacher's expectations that she could make this inference and work that out for herself. Without the diagnosis of AS I fear at this point I would be receiving reports of 'lack of common sense' at the very best, 'stupid' at the worst. Instead, I feel that this episode serves to demonstrate to teaching staff the need to be explicit in their instructions and will have heightened their awareness of some of the difficulties in communicating with someone with AS, perhaps becoming more attentive to their *own* language, rather than focusing on the pupil's.

It is a big step, sharing the news of Eva's diagnosis with a wider population via this book, but I want us to be bold about being an 'ally for Asperger's'. I like the word 'ally', especially the definition in the dictionary that says it means to 'Combine or unite a resource (with another) for mutual benefit'. Telling a wider audience about Eva's Asperger's is a step we have decided on together, and although she's a young person to make a decision like this, she has her own mind, has her own opinions and wants to be accepted for who she is. Perhaps for this reason, Eva has never been particularly interested in making relationships (real or in cyberspace) with other people with AS although she's not avoiding it; her life is too busy and there are too many other people in her immediate world that she is interested in spending time with. There are lots of forums on the internet for people with AS to get together and that's got to be a good thing; it's just something Eva hasn't got into at this point, perhaps never will. It's up to her what she does with the information as she gets older. The internet chat rooms that refer to individuals as 'Aspies' are the ones *I* avoid as I don't think it's helpful to identify anyone by a genetic or neurological feature. To do so is to ignore the lovely, beautiful array of individuality we can see in people with AS and ASD. Imagine, for example, if we began to call left-handed people 'lefties' and right-handed people 'righties'. It has positive and negative connotations for both groups of people and does not describe the wide range of personalities, skills, problems, abilities, talents, deficits or anything else about a group of people. All it does is encourage the rest of the world to stereotype individuals according to a neurological feature. I'm nervous about reactions to the book, but not about reactions to Eva as a person with AS; we have lovely friends and family that love us so what more could

I ask for? On an interesting note, Eva never did get round to telling anyone in her school year (staff or pupils) during a year in Australia that she had AS – this wasn't avoidance, it was just more relevant to say she was *English* and had just moved continents. An end of year email from the Vice Principal in the school told me: 'She (Eva) would be an asset to any school.' Moved me to tears, that did, and especially so because it was a comment about Eva as a person, not as a person with a label or disability.

Eva (15 years)

As far I know most people perceive autism as a bad thing but there's a programme on TV called 'The Big Bang Theory' that has a central character called Sheldon who is hilarious and it seems like he has AS to me...he's somebody I suspect has AS because he's really logical, he hasn't got great social skills and is definitely above average intelligence and has obsessions about certain things. He struggles being interested in things that other people are interested in because to him, *his* interests are more fascinating (like Leonard Nimoy (Spock from Star Trek) for example). Sheldon has particular habits and ways of doing things that he has to stick to. I guess he's a stereotype of someone with AS but he's really great because he always gets things just how he likes them, is really organised and is fixed enough on his goals that he always achieves them. He's got a PhD and is successful in his job as a theoretical physicist. The reason I introduced him here is because he's a hugely popular comedy figure with AS that has lots of successes (even if they're fictional ones!); friends, work, a girlfriend...plus he's totally loveable. He gets annoyed when people interrupt him but he has to keep talking about his own thing, or when something changes in his routine and I'm a bit like that... I might not look like we behave the same way but often on the inside I'm doing exactly what he's doing.

I guess what I'm trying to say is that stereotypes are a dangerous thing because they lead to people making assumptions and being blinded to who you really are, who I really am and anything positive about me.

I told my closest friends that I had AS when I first got diagnosed, and like I said earlier, they weren't really interested. I think they didn't know anything about AS and saw autism as a disability that they didn't recognise in me. It's never been anything we talked about, then or now and I don't really know why. If anyone treated me differently because of my diagnosis either I didn't notice or I can't remember because it wasn't significant.

CHAPTER 11

Strategies
That Help

or 'you have stepped unknowingly in a massive pile of poo'

My Asperger's hero Tony Attwood wrote a paper about how children with Asperger's 'actively look for friendship but in a clumsy and not very successful way'.[7] This is so, so true of Eva who has always wanted to 'connect' with other children but, until recently, found it so hard because of her aforementioned style of interaction, communication and social functioning. There are things I have done with Eva just because I'm her mum, and things I have taken a sort of strategic approach to because she has always appeared to be wired slightly differently from other kids and I think it's good to think about the things that you *want* to do and provide your child with as a parent; these things reflect your values and your beliefs...but there are also things that your child *needs* because they are not neurotypical.

What I want to do in this chapter is rattle on about the things that I have made a conscious effort to do, because I could see where there were things that Eva found difficult, or things that made others react to her in a negative way. None of them require any skills other than that of loving her and being a parent that knows her own child although I must admit that I sometimes feel slightly guilty that I tried to be her therapist at times, rather than her Mother. I must say, we have had loads of fun with all of this, lots of fantastic games and conversations and real 'quality time' with my beautiful daughter. Eva absolutely has always known her own mind and if I ever got it wrong (which I continue to do) or introduced an idea that she just wasn't interested in, I have respected that and said 'OK – let's forget it and I'll take the dog for a walk instead.' (Great thing, having a dog – they do so put up with grumpiness and mine has been a great role model and taught me fabulous stuff like never passing up the opportunity to go for a joyride, taking little naps, *always* being pleased to see a familiar face and to greet them with enthusiasm, and when you're happy to wiggle your whole body in a joyful dance! We all have so much to learn and young people with AS are smart enough to know that too. I absolutely believe that parents are the best teachers for their children.

Help young people with AS by giving them opportunities to interact with other children

For my sanity (and hers!) I have always tried very hard to give Eva opportunities to interact with neurotypical children. This is really important because young people with AS can be a whizz at 'lifting' behaviours and scripts that they have seen elsewhere (including on TV but also from other children) and using these behaviours and scripts as if they were their own. This sounds like it is something neurotypical children do, but the rigidity and repetitiveness of how children with AS do this is what makes it different. Don't be fooled! These young people have a whole host of strategies they use like a smoke-screen to hide the fact that they actually don't know how to behave in a group or in a conversation and if you listen carefully and long enough you will begin to realise that the conversation they are having was something you watched on 'Doctor Who' last Saturday, or a game they are playing was something you saw Bart Simpson do last week. And they will repeat the whole thing again and again and in different situations because it 'worked' for them last time – they have no strategies to adapt their communication or behaviour when the next situation is different. There was never any doubt in my mind that Eva wouldn't attend a mainstream school; that was the obvious choice but I always bore in mind that unstructured 'play' times can be hell for young people with AS who will find it hard to be in a large group. Think of the chaos, noise and free for all in the playground! All those mini people running around like headless chickens, shouting and screaming – and what are the rules at playtime? There aren't any! So it's very hard for kids with AS to know what to 'do' at playtime. I always encouraged her to join clubs and activities that the school put on at break times, like choir practice or dance club. In high school, she became a volunteer in the school library at lunch time which gave her a specific role to play.

When she was younger, Eva was a genius at finding *one* person (usually someone quiet and compliant) and leading them into her imaginary world. I actively encouraged this imaginary world (it even had its own language) and helped Eva to build fantasies about it that she and her friend could then enact in the playground. So I guess what I'm saying is don't be afraid to give your child a 'script' because kids with AS are fantastic at memorising lines and imitating so they make pretty good 'actors' at an early age. Other opportunities for being with other kids really needed to be structured – having someone round to the house to 'play' was stressful for Eva, me and probably the other child too. Weekends Eva went to Stagecoach (dance, music, theatre group) and I have to say that Cery and James, the Stagecoach leaders in her school, were the best thing that could have happened to her – they gave her loads of structure, loads of direction about what to 'do' and always, always were massively positive about her and *to* her. She loves them. She really does, even though she no longer goes there. Any other groups that have planned activities or a specific focus (like dance classes, Cubs and Brownies) will provide kids with AS with the clear direction they need, and the opportunity to practise interacting in a group.

Help young people with AS by teaching them about Asperger's Syndrome and being positive about it

I think things really started to change for Eva after she got diagnosed – that is why we both advocate so strongly for assessment. Knowing and understanding yourself and having a name for it is a fantastic starting block for any young person to choose what they would like to change about themselves. For Eva, there were definitely some physical behaviours that she could very quickly see were what people called 'weird'. These included (amongst others) flapping her arms, twiddling her fingers in front of her face, not making good eye contact and pulling goofy faces. If you have ever tried to change your *own* behaviour in some way (think diets, stopping smoking, etc.) can you remember what you replaced your previous behaviour with? We are almost always successful if we have an alternative to the thing we want to 'give up.' Just *stopping doing it* is really hard without a replacement activity – so think about the behaviour you would like to change, and plan an alternative one. Then act it out. Then think of one time or place you could do that in.

Getting anywhere yet? So for Eva to stop pulling goofy faces when she saw someone she knew, she had practised an alternative to that by saying 'Hi – how are you?' at home with me, many times, before she decided that she was going to say it to her friend A, next time she saw her. I can't remember if she came up with the words, or was it me? I think it is perfectly fine to have given her a script! And once she had been successful doing it for that first time, successive attempts to do it got easier and easier.

Help young people with AS by helping them to develop positive self-esteem

Even if there is *nothing* the young person wants to change about themselves, I still believe it is important to know about Asperger's and have a name for what is hard in their life. These are not stupid people – people with AS have average or above-average intellectual abilities so they will not fail to notice if people avoid them, or leave them out of things, or walk away from a conversation with them. I'm going to wander off on a bit of a tangent here for a moment; please bear with me while I try to find an analogy that will explain what I mean... Imagine, for a moment, that you have stepped unknowingly in a massive and foul-smelling pile of poo but that a bad cold renders you incapable of detecting the odour. As you approach people they back away in horror or start wafting their hands in front of their noses. You see this and you *know* there is something 'wrong' with you but have no way of detecting the problem. It seems like the problem is *you* and you have no way to fix it. If you knew it wasn't you but, in fact, the dog poo on your shoe you could quickly nip out and clean your shoes off on the lawn. Now I feel really guilty that I chose such a ridiculous analogy and maybe it's a bit insulting too, to compare AS to a pile of dog poo (for which I make a grovelling apology for my lack of inventiveness with analogy), but the point I am trying to make is that kids with AS can tell that relationships or interactions break down, but if they don't have a name for it, or an understanding of what that is, then the only other possible explanation is that there is something *wrong* with them. This is why so many young people with AS end up with secondary diagnoses of clinical depression or other mood disorders.

Eva is rightly proud of having Asperger's and can make decisions about the bits she wants to 'keep' and the things she is prepared to move on. For example, she knows it is limiting and inconvenient and just plain awkward to insist on a restrictive diet that meets her sensory preferences. Going out for dinner, or eating at a friend's house, can be 'embarrassing' if you're really fussy about what's on your plate or how it is served. Therefore she is prepared to 'try' new foods and how they are combined and in this way she has, over the years, gone from a fish-fingers-and-chips girl to a teenager that can order her own food in a restaurant and say how she would like it served ('Steak cooked medium rare but with *no* onions or sauce on it please'). My final comment in this section is that I love it when Eva says 'Nooooooo! You have to let me be autistic about this!' Anybody with that level of clarity deserves respect I think.

Help young people with AS by teaching 'Theory of Mind' skills

There are plenty of books and programmes of work that are designed for professionals to use with children with AS and ASD to help them in understanding what other people are thinking or doing – for example, Carol Gray's *Comic Strip Conversations*[8] and Patricia Howlin, Simon Baron-Cohen and Julie Hadwin's *Teaching Children with Autism to Mind-Read*[9] but these are designed for a very broad population and the professionals working with your child may not know exactly what kind of difficulties s/he is having with developing Theory of Mind. They focus on how to interpret facial expressions or to recognise the different feelings of anger, sadness, fear and happiness. They are also aiming to help young people to see things from another person's perspective, and how to understand another person's knowledge and beliefs. I think it is incredibly hard to teach young people emotional understanding from a set of pictures or photographs. For example, a look of terror on someone's face isn't a static thing, and it's usually accompanied by a scream or frightened words. When we are happy, we don't have a great big goofy happy grin permanently on our faces – we may laugh momentarily and talk in an upbeat way... but does a photo of a smiling person labelled 'Happy' teach us that someone who is *not* smiling fixedly is *un*happy? Emotions are shown by a series of very rapid facial expressions so using photos to explain emotions in others is not always helpful. I have found it much more useful to help Eva develop Theory of Mind, including an understanding of emotions, by playing a sort of 'Explanations game' with her. We've never given it a name as such, it's something we have developed unspoken just through our conversations, but it goes something like this.

Eva tells me something that happened at school and I aim to get her to come up with explanations for what's happened. The explanations fall into four categories:

- *psychological explanations* ('She stayed in at lunch time *because she wanted to*')

- *physical explanations* ('She stayed in at lunch time *because she was hungry and was eating her lunch*')

- *conventional explanations* (explanations about rules and conventions, such as 'she stayed in at lunch time *because she had a detention*')

- *biological explanations* ('She stayed in *because she was sick*').

Figuring out these explanations needs an adult (me!) to ask lots of questions and to model (give examples of) other explanations. What I was aiming for was to help Eva to see a different perspective from her own. Explaining someone else's more advanced reasoning or motives challenges a young person's current understanding and stretches her understanding about what and why people think and feel what they do. I must say, at this point in Eva's life, and for the past couple of years, I am no longer the person asking the questions but Eva is asking questions and seeking explanations for herself. She is so adept at this now I would say that arguably she has greater emotional literacy skills than the majority of her class mates, analyses and explains other people's perspectives and shows great empathy, especially with her friends' boyfriend-related problems!

Just bear in mind that Theory of Mind is something that usually starts early in life but continues to develop throughout life – there's no end point!

Help young people with AS by teaching them conversation skills

Having successful conversations is so dependent on who you are talking to – this is true of everyone, not just something that some people with AS find challenging. Conversation needs so many skills:

paying attention, processing information, interpreting and understanding vocabulary, even before you start taking conversation 'turns' or contributing your own ideas and opinions. Conversations are also very unpredictable and change quickly as well as there being different 'rules' to conversation dependent on who you are talking to. However, there are some basic conversation 'skills' and 'rules' that you can help young people with AS to learn.

Conversation starters – Give your young person a script: great ways to start conversations include *questions* ('How are you?' / 'What have you been up to?' / 'Did you see Doctor Who last night?'), *compliments* ('You look nice' / 'I like your jacket' / 'You have beautiful eyes') and *friendly comments* ('It's a nice day' / 'I can't wait 'til lunch time'). Telling a young person with AS that they can use these three things (Questions, Compliments, Friendly Comments) and giving examples of these can help them to learn a bit of a script to strike up conversations with others. I know I keep saying it, but having a 'script' is something that we all do to some extent; if you meet the public in your working life, don't you have a pre-practised set of 'lines' that you use? 'Are you looking for anything in particular?' or 'How can I help you?' or 'Suits you Sir!' There is no reason that young people can't be provided with the script...where the conversation leads to and how it develops is *all* outside of our control; it's dependent on so many different factors. I always worked hard at getting Eva to start conversations and she's truly great at it now – I hear her strike up conversations with loads of different people with 'So what have you been up to?' And 'I love the snow!' and a squillion other phrases... the days of awkward silences are over.

Conversation rules – Standing the right distance from your conversation 'partner' is relatively easy; often young people with AS love this 'rule' because it's sort of scientific and measurable. You only have to explain it, show it and then ask them to make sure that's what they're doing...a generalisation here, because it *does* depend on who you're talking to, but half an arm's length is close enough for the person to know that you are talking to them but not so close that you're 'in their face'. It's also helpful to tell someone to observe in a group situation how close all the other people are to each other. Also notice if you move closer to someone and they back away – you're probably just a little bit too much in their personal space and should step back a little. This is something you can practise at home.

Eye contact is, I think, a contentious issue. Some people make more eye contact than others naturally but as a very broad rule we tend to keep eye contact 60–70 per cent of the time in general conversation. Staring intently at people results in the other person feeling like they've got something wrong with them, or can be an aggressive stance and what we want to do in conversation with others is to give them a feeling of comfort of warm interest in what they are saying. I don't think it's worth trying to 'teach' eye contact...just talking about it with someone with AS is useful; it's good to raise awareness and help them to work out how other people might feel as a result of their behaviour.

Topic maintenance – This refers to flexibly using a style of speech suited to the situation and conversational partners, and working out what information will be relevant and interesting to others. We all love to go on (and on!) about our favourite topics (especially me – I am already nearly at the end of a book) but we generally consider and adapt our conversation to be of interest to other people. This can be really hard for young people with AS who often have a subject that is very dear to their hearts, something that they know about in great detail and that they like to talk about at length. It's also hard for them to summarise or pick out the important or most significant features of a subject so they can tend to have to tell you *all* the details when just one or two key points would have done the job. Teaching topic maintenance is a real challenge that you can start by getting a person with AS to *identify* what the topic is, and to look out for topic 'clues' in what the other person says. It's not rocket science – you just have to watch TV together or a favourite film and stop from time to time to ask 'what were they talking about?' Ask if they can tell you the answer using just *one* word, rather than having them recite the whole dialogue back at you – once the young person has become skilled at identifying topics in this way you can move on to shifting a conversation to include another topic, and ask them did they spot the 'clue' you were giving them to talk about something else.

Help young people with AS by teaching organisation skills

When Eva started high school her first term was a mass of detentions for not doing her homework and not having the right books or equipment and the best thing I did, when I discovered how poorly organised she was at school, was to print off her timetable and stick it in the hallway next to the shelf where she dumped her school bag when she came in. She only needed a small prompt 'Get your bag ready for the morning' from me every evening and she could stand in the hall, *look* at her timetable and work out what books and other things she needed to put in her bag. Most young people with ASD or AS have poor organisational skills and this one was amongst a couple of things that I could do to help her organise herself independently as well as discovering some new things that I hadn't even considered. One of these surprises was that she never wrote in her school 'planner', the diary that is given to all high school students to note down assignments and events in their week. I asked Eva why she didn't have much written in it and she told me that she didn't know what to write...that couldn't be right! It took almost three terms before I discovered that when she got into a classroom her planner never left her bag! She didn't like the 'feel' of it (it had a funny textured cover on it – read my chapter about sensory integration!) and so it stayed in her bag. No wonder she never did any homework – she wasn't writing it down and her memory isn't *that* amazing. Once we worked this out, I put a clear plastic, smooth cover on the planner and simply told her to take it out of her bag whenever she took her pencil case out...it's still not her greatest skill but so much improved from that first muddle of a year.

Young people with AS often appear disorganised and that can be as a result of not understanding what has been said, or not being able to work out what is expected of them. So what we need to do is establish *routines* that help them to become 'organised'. Routines are great for all of us, especially for people with AS. Routines mean that we can predict what will happen, we know how to behave and we generally understand the consequences when routines aren't stuck to. Lots of routines can start off with 'rules'; things that an adult imposes on a child but we want our young people to do things independently so we don't have to be watching them all of the time and telling them what to do. Rules, when we stick to them, quickly turn into routine behaviours that children can do for themselves and this is what I aimed for whenever I set a new rule for Eva. So we had a 'rule' about hanging her bag up in the hallway (next to her timetable!), a rule for setting out her clothes the night before, a rule for brushing her teeth for three minutes at a time, etc. I think the important thing to do is *say* what the rule is, and make sure you give a visual clue too – after all, a spoken instruction lasts a very short time, but a visual clue is there constantly so it helps to hear and see what is expected from you at the same time.

I gave Eva visual reminders to help her stick to the rules. Her timetable on the wall was a visual reminder, so was her toothbrush timer stuck on the bathroom wall. (You can get these online very cheaply – some of them are simple, low-tech ones that look a bit like an old-fashioned egg-timer with sand that runs from one bit to another but ours is a battery-operated, stick-on-the-wall one with a light-up display that you press when you start brushing your teeth and flashes red after three minutes.)

You can also use 'Visual Timetables' to help establish routines at home and for ones that are school-related. This is just a timetable featuring days of the week or hours of the day and means that the young person can easily see what activities they need to be doing at that time. You can write down words, or make one with pictures or photos and stick them up in appropriate places – so for example if you want to help a young person keep their bedroom organised, make a timetable that you stick on the bedroom door that has 'hang clothes up', 'put books away', 'make bed' and then *finally* 'play on laptop'. This way, they are able to see the order in which they need to do things and this saves lots of shouting matches and unclear, muttered comments from you about their room 'looking like a pig-sty', which, for someone with AS, is a totally confusing comment – it has no pigs in it and isn't a request to do anything about it anyway!

Every year in school, tasks become more complex, the organisational demands increase, and children are given greater responsibility for monitoring their behaviour and working independently. Eva has a load of routines now that she uses in and around the home but sometimes finds it hard to organise her school work. I have given Eva 'writing frames' to help her complete her homework in an organised way; a writing frame is a list of what you need to write about and in what order. I'm going to go off at a small tangent here to try and illustrate what I mean. Did you ever play that game 'Consequences' when you were at school? The one where you have a piece of paper on which to write and then you fold it over to conceal what you've written and hand it to the next person in a group to write the next bit of a story? It went something like this:

- a boy's name and they met...

- a girl's name

- where they met

- what they did

- what she said

- what he said

- what happened in the end (the consequence).

After everyone had completed it, you could unfold the bit of paper to read out a nonsensical 'story' such as 'Mickey Mouse met'…'Kate Middleton'….'in Primark' and 'they flew to outer space'…she said 'A large burger and a regular fries please'…he said 'That's what makes you beautiful'…and in the end they 'became a huge YouTube sensation'.

I have to confess to enormously enjoying making that up by texting the questions to my various friends as I write – they have no idea what I'm doing but are happy to go along with the questions as I ask them! I really *am* trying to illustrate the point of giving a writing frame to someone so will return to the matter in hand: a writing frame sets out the points that need to be made which provides someone with AS with clues about what to include or not include in a written piece of work. So a writing frame to complete a history assignment, for example, might be a sheet of paper with the following headings on:

- Research and gather information about the Romans.

- What happened to people in the UK?

- Why did it happen?

- What problems were there?

- What solutions were there?

- What is your opinion about this?

Writing frames take many forms and there are lots of resources on-line and available from schools or you can make your own. When Eva starts a piece of written work now, she often creates her own 'frame', which is a series of questions she thinks need answering. It's not unlike how people write reports using different headings to make sure that they cover all the necessary information.

There are so many different aspects to AS and we must not forget that all people with AS or ASD are totally individual, so what 'works' for one person will not necessarily work for another. Still, I believe that these are areas of difficulty that are common to all people with AS: interacting with others, understanding themselves and other people, maintaining self-esteem, conversation skills and organising themselves and their lives independently... after all, these are the criteria that define someone as having AS. They aren't areas that are exclusive to AS. They just don't occur all together in other people like they do with AS. Finally, I really, really believe that *all* young people need a whole army of allies, to help them develop and reach their potential...the more people we have supporting young people with AS in a multitude of ways, the better, I say.

Eva (15 years)

If I had a magic wand I'd cast a spell on my teachers to ensure that I was listening to them, paying attention and understanding what is going on in all of my classes without them unintentionally embarrassing me by 'checking' that I've got the message. In some classes I don't need the teachers to check with me, like English where I'm really stimulated and there are always visual materials like PowerPoint presentations. I can take in this info and listen and write at the same time. With other classes, as long as I am sitting with friends I can check with them but when I'm just listening to someone, I find it hard to focus my attention. With science, there are lots of mathematical and chemical equations that I find hard even though there are lots of 'rules' about how to work things out. I know that teachers' intentions are to make sure that I know what's going on, and I appreciate that they are trying to help me but asking 'Have you got that, Eva?' is totally embarrassing and pointless 'cause when I *do* get it, I don't need them to check and when I *haven't* got it, I'm not going to embarrass myself by saying out loud 'Uh – no, actually.' If I felt OK about admitting to that I would have asked for help in the first place! I need to learn to not be so self-conscious, rather than my teachers having to do something different for me.

Understanding what AS is is the one thing that has had a hugely positive effect on my life. I don't know many people with AS but the things that other people with AS report that you read on the internet and see on YouTube aren't very positive... I think I've been properly educated about AS and I know what I need to do in order to make my life easier. I don't think I have needed to change much, just needed to know more about myself and I guess I've been learning about AS from an early age. I know that I'm not neurotypical but that's OK and I know the things I need to question about myself, like have I really considered other people's points of view which I've got really good at now and am constantly trying to do it. I also know when I *don't* understand a scenario enough to be able to put myself in someone else's shoes and understand it from their point of view so I think I'm getting more aware.

My biology teacher thinks I'm uber-smart because I use terminology in class, in casual conversation, about atypical and neurotypical behaviours... actually it's really helped to have this vocabulary to describe myself and other people and differences between us. I'm a word person so it's great to have terminology to choose from.

I've never been discriminated against by friends or in school as far as I know, and I'm happy that I'm accepted for being myself, not for someone with AS. I don't need anyone to treat me like I'm special or go out of their way to treat me differently...it has been brilliant that school are sensitive and aware that sometimes I get in a muddle or need to be told things in a different way. The most important strategy to be used around people with AS is to treat them as individuals, as opposed to someone with stereotyped needs.

CHAPTER 12

Asperger's Syndrome

or 'I'm the last of my kind'

In May 2013, the labelling of different degrees of autism in children and adults changed. The fifth edition of the *Diagnostic and Statistical Manual of Mental Disorders* (DSM-5) abandoned the terms 'autistic disorder', 'Asperger's syndrome', 'childhood disintegrative disorder' and 'PDD-NOS' (pervasive developmental disorder – not otherwise specified), instead classing them together under a single diagnosis: 'autism spectrum disorders'.

The 'old' criteria for AS and ASD were grouped into three areas of difficulties (1.social interaction, 2.social communication, 3.restricted repetitive behaviours). The new criteria have just two categories: 1. social communication and interaction,

2. restricted, repetitive patterns of behaviour, interests or activities (which includes sensory behaviours and preferences).

The DSM-5 claims to change the emphasis from 'labelling' a condition to identifying individuals' needs and being specific about how much support they will need. For that reason three levels of need for each of the two areas of difficulty have been introduced:

- Level 1 - requiring support.

- Level 2 - requiring substantial support.

- Level 3 - requiring very substantial support.

The only problem with this is that 'support' varies from region to region so what is available in one town or city isn't necessarily on offer somewhere else. Likewise what is classed as 'substantial' or 'very substantial' may be different in different regions. There is also the risk that making a diagnosis directly linked to levels of support may influence the professionals making the decisions.

The National Autistic Society have got lots of really good points of view and information about this so their website is well worth reading. What pleases me particularly is that they have campaigned for much more attention to be given to assessment and diagnosis of girls and women with autism as they feel these may be under-diagnosed. I think girls don't fit the (male) autistic stereotype – look at what my daughter Rosy said about this! – so perhaps autism stays 'under the radar' more in girls, and they are not referred for assessment as often as they should be. It would be interesting to look at numbers of girls referred for assessment compared to boys.

If I had one wish, it would be that there was an extra level below 'requiring support' called 'requiring awareness'. This is what I really want: for people with AS or ASD to have lots of opportunities (like Eva) to become more self-aware – as well as other people, society as a whole, not just teachers and other professionals, to be more aware of people who are not neurotypical. I don't think 'support' is necessarily the best word to describe how people with AS need other people to change their attitudes. Isn't that the biggest challenge, really? For autism to not always be viewed as a 'problem' or disability? I once asked Eva what she thought about telling other kids about having AS and she said the problem with it was that it was called a 'syndrome' and that sounded like someone with 'special needs', someone who had problems generally and therefore other people would have preconceived ideas about what she was like. I think, for us, raising awareness of 'differences' rather than 'difficulties' might compare to how the deaf community view deafness – they see it as a difference in human condition rather than a disability. I can get that.

The other issue I have is with the label 'Asperger's Syndrome' in the first place. I think for some it has been a much more positive term than autism and that in some cases children and parents can use the term Asperger's to suggest intellectual superiority whereas 'autism' always implies something negative, a deficit of some sort. Perhaps using ASD as a wider term will do something towards challenging society's stereotypes and help people think of those with ASD more individually...only time can tell. I asked Eva what she thought about 'Asperger's' not being a diagnostic term any more and she, always the joker, said 'I'm cured!'

Eva (15 years)

I have never referred to myself as 'an Aspie'. Firstly because I hate the word (it sounds like a form of parasite), but also I've never heard anyone describe *themselves* with that term in a positive way. Having labels for things can be useful at times – but if you say 'Autism' to people they think 'special needs' or 'learning disability' whereas when you say 'Asperger's' they often have more positive associations. I suppose this might be because it's less well known that the people who *do* know about AS are more likely to understand it properly. I prefer to describe myself as someone whose brain is wired differently, or someone who is not neurotypical and I don't mind being thought of as autistic. I suppose the changes to the DSM 'labels' are a good thing 'cause people won't be able to stereotype Autism the way they have in the past. It's gonna take time...

CHAPTER 13

The Present and the Future

or 'not barking like a dog'

So I started writing this book in 2010 soon after Eva received a diagnosis, and boy-oh-boy have things changed since then. Eva is incredible at 15 years old; I have taken her around the world, moved to Australia for a year where she attended a local high school and reinvented herself. The reinvention had already begun before we moved though, and that is why we made it to Australia. That first year of high school in the UK was a muddle of Eva in trouble for non-completion or submission of homework, or not having the right equipment for school on the right days, or being confused about her friendships. Her teachers said she 'didn't listen' and were, at times, frustrated by her random comments and ability to talk at length about something that appeared to them as irrelevant. She made some new friends and fell out with some old ones. For the first time in her life, she had a (small) group of girlies to hang out with. By the time she turned 14 (living in Melbourne at the time) she had perfected the art of 'hanging out with her girlies' and if anyone ever thought she was 'weird' they probably put it down to her being from the UK.

When I 'liked' a friend's comment on Facebook about working in Australia, little did I think Eva would be the one egging me on to go, making me stay there the first three months that were incredibly hard on me as an individual and professionally. She really kept me going with her rigidity; we had said we were going to go, so we *had* to (in spite of the challenge of visa applications, having nowhere to live when we got there, not enough money to travel, finding a foster home for the dog for a year and the wrench of leaving my gorgeous old dad and my older daughter behind). Professionals would say it was autistic rigidity; I have a friend who says it is 'Providence'.[10] And we are back in the UK after a whole year in Australia. Eva was fine during our time there; she had lots of Australian girlies to hang with and nobody called her weird except me, now and again. She can get to call me names too if she likes ('idiot' features heavily in her vocabulary when she's addressing me and she's right, I often *am* an idiot and do idiotic things that probably seem completely irrational to her logical approach to life). She continues to be fantastic now we are home and in her new school, as I mentioned earlier.

Eva has grown (she'll hate me for saying this) in stature (now towers over her 'big' sister and can see eye to eye with me (ha ha) but it is nothing in comparison to how she has grown in terms of her social and communicative development. We have had some funny times that have got us to this point. Last year, in the car, I sort of sensed her looking at me while I was driving and I became self-conscious and asked what she was looking at. Did I have a bogey on my face or something? Grown another head? (Or only yet another chin?) 'Duh! I'm doing eye contact (idiot)' she replied.

Hmmm. Driving down the motorway is perhaps not the best place to practise eye contact, but still... It demonstrated an awareness of herself, what she was doing that she could articulate clearly and rationally. *This* is what having a diagnosis of Asperger's has meant to Eva – she has been able to learn about social and communication behaviours and skills, and make an active decision about the ones she wants to improve upon.

As far as I am concerned, Eva is the best 14 year old in both Northern and Southern hemispheres. Perhaps a bit shy sometimes, but not always. Sometimes awkward, but hey, isn't that 15? I still question what she is thinking and doing too much, overanalyse and often get it wrong. I don't mind her telling me that I am 'patronising' or just 'wrong' and content with being told I am, as it stimulates debate and discussion between us.

I have become increasingly aware of a number of fictional works with characters in them with AS or ASD (*The Curious Incident of the Dog in the Night-Time*[11], *The Way Things Look to Me*[12], *House Rules*[13], *The Boy Who Fell to Earth*[14]) that are all in the public domain and make for popular reading. I think that, on the whole, these can be no bad thing, and that they are raising the awareness of AS but I really long for a book or a film about someone with AS that just functions in the world without barking like a dog, being a child-genius or planning their own death or that of someone else with military precision. So many people I know say 'I'm being a bit autistic' when what they are actually trying to say is 'I am feeling rigid and inflexible and I like my dishwasher stacked like this.' I do so wish they would say *that* instead of mislabelling autism. Or those people that describe someone else as 'a bit Aspergie' or something akin to that to describe someone who is socially awkward. Let us get it right for our children and young people and don't underestimate autism. Being inflexible isn't what makes someone autistic or have AS; there is so much more to this complex condition.

I hope this book has introduced you to a lovely 15-year-old girl and helped you think about the good things about having a diagnosis of AS. It would be good for the world to see how 'ordinary' Eva is in many ways – she's not having a meltdown in the supermarket because the vegetables aren't lined up in alphabetical order, and Eva doesn't only eat foods beginning with 'm' on Monday, 't' on Tuesday. She is interested in boys and clothes and music and theatre and photography and makeup and is obsessive about her hair (15! – that's all). She doesn't need to have any extra help in school…sometimes she misses out on doing something or gets in trouble for not doing a piece of work like any other teenager. My theory is that she has zoned out or that she has become distracted with sensory integration issues when being told something. She'll tell you that she just 'forgot.' Her teachers will tell you she doesn't listen. Whatever. I can look at her and categorise the elements that make her a young woman with Asperger's but that's not who she *is*. She is just who she is, not identifiable by a diagnosis. And it certainly isn't a disability in the general understanding of that word, in spite of the World Health Organisation classification. If you want to think about this statement a bit more, or disagree strongly, read experts like Wendy Lawson who says 'There has never been a better time to be autistic'[15] and I believe she is right. With people like her, many others and young people like Eva advocating for autism, Asperger's or whatever you, or they want to call it, our world gets to be a better, more tolerant and ultimately more intelligent and lovely place to be.

Endnotes

1. Attwood, T. (2013) *The Pattern of Abilities and Development of Girls with Asperger's Syndrome*. Available at www.tonyattwood.com. au/index.php/publications/by-tony-attwood/archived-papers/80-the-pattern-of-abilities-and-development-of-girls-with-aspergers-syndrome, accessed on 24 April 2014.

2. Jackson, L. (2002) *Freaks, Geeks and Asperger Syndrome: A User Guide to Adolescence*. London: Jessica Kingsley Publishers.

3. 'Asperger's syndrome is mostly a "hidden disability". This means that you can't tell that someone has the condition from their outward appearance. People with the condition have difficulties in three main areas. They are:

    - social communication
    - social interaction
    - social imagination.

    They are often referred to as "the triad of impairments". While there are similarities with autism, people with Asperger's syndrome have fewer problems with speaking and are often of average, or above average, intelligence. They do not usually have the accompanying learning disabilities associated with autism, but they may have specific learning difficulties. These may include dyslexia and dyspraxia or other conditions such as attention deficit hyperactivity disorder (ADHD) and epilepsy.'

(From The National Autistic Society (2014) 'What is Asperger Syndrome?' Available at www.autism.org.uk/about-autism/ autism-and-asperger-syndrome-an-introduction/what-is-asperger-syndrome.aspx, accessed 14 February 2014)

4. American Psychiatric Association (2013) 'Hightlights of Changes from DSM-IV-TR to DSM-5.' Available at http://www.dsm5.org/ Documents/changes%20from%20dsm-iv-tr%20to%20dsm-5.pdf, accessed on 27 April 2014.

5. Baron-Cohen, S. (2001) 'Theory of mind in normal development and autism.' *Prisme 34*, 174–183.

6. http://www.mind.org.uk/information-support/types-of-mental-health-problems/obsessive-compulsive-disorder-(ocd)/#U3ip-_ ldX1

7. Attwood, T. (2013) *Strategies for Improving the Social Integration of Children with Asperger's Syndrome*. Available at www.tonyattwood. com.au/index.php?option=com_content&view=article&id= 72:strategies-for-improving-the-social-integration-of-children-with-aspergers-syndrome&catid=45:archived-resource-papers&-Itemid=181, accessed on 27 April 2014.

8. Gray, C. (1994) *Comic Strip Conversations: Illustrated Interactions that Teach Conversation Skills to Students with Autism and Related Disorders*. Arlington, TX: Future Horizons Incorporated.

9. Howlin, P., Baron-Cohen, S. and Hadwin, J. (1998) *Teaching Children with Autism to Mind-Read*. Chichester: John Wiley & Sons.

10. 'Until one is committed, there is hesitancy, the chance to draw back – Concerning all acts of initiative (and creation), there is one elementary truth that ignorance of which kills countless ideas and splendid plans: that the moment one definitely commits oneself, then Providence moves too. All sorts of things occur to help one that would never otherwise have occurred. A whole stream of events issues from the decision, raising in one's favor all manner of unforeseen incidents and meetings and material assistance, which no man could have dreamed would have come his way. Whatever you can do, or dream you can do, begin it. Boldness has genius, power, and magic in it. Begin it now.' William Hutchinson Murray. (1951) *The Scottish Himalayan Expedition*. London: Dent.

11. Haddon, M. (2003) *The Curious Incident of the Dog in the Night-Time*. London: Jonathan Cape.

12. Farooki, R. (2009) *The Way Things Look to Me*. London: Pan Books.

13. Piccoult, J. (2010) *House Rules*. London: Hodder & Stoughton.

14. Lette, K. (2012) *The Boy Who Fell to Earth*. London: Transworld Publishers.

15. Lawson, W. (2012) 'An Introduction to Dr. Wendy Lawson.' Available at www.mugsy.org/wendy/tour.htm, accessed on 28 April 2014.

Index

American Psychiatric
Association (APA)
11
AS see Asperger's
Syndrome
ASD see Autistic
Spectrum Disorders
Asperger's Syndrome
(AS)
assessment see
assessments for
ASD
being an 'ally for
Asperger's' 86–7
being different 17–23,
41–4, 80
being ordinary
120–21
being positive about
19, 85, 94, 95–6,
110–11, 115–16
diagnosis see diagnosis
of Asperger's
Syndrome/ASD
DSM-5 categories of
support levels 114,
115
DSM-5 change to
autism spectrum
conditions 11–12,
113–14, 116
and family
relationships
75–82, 92

and fitting in 18–19,
22–4
and food 64, 78, 97–8
friendship-seeking by
people with 91
and gender 21–2,
114–15
having, not suffering
from 23–4
helping children with
AS think about
themselves 18–20
and labelling 17–19,
83–4, 113–14,
115–16
and language see
language
online forums for
people with 87
and organisation skills
104–9
and parental blame 31
providing child
interaction
opportunities for
young people with
93–5
public awareness
raised through
fictional characters
120
repetitive behaviours
with see repetitive
behaviours
and school see schools

and self-awareness
18–19, 22–4, 33,
119
and self-esteem 20,
21, 96–8, 109
sensory integration
difficulties 57–67
and social skills
see social/
communication
skills
stereotypes 43, 70,
79–80, 88–9
strategies that help
people with
91–112
talking to a child
about 19–20, 21,
22, 31–2, 95–6
and Theory of Mind
52–4, 98–100
assessments for ASD
assessment team
members 25
deciding on
assessment 17–24
getting an assessment
25–33
getting a diagnosis
13–16, 25–6, 28
play-based 29–30
school involvement in
30–31
talking to a child
about 21

126

INDEX

Lightning Source UK Ltd.
Milton Keynes UK
UKOW03f0026230714

235598UK00001B/10/P